United Cerebral Palsy
2141 Overlook
Rd.
44106

DEVELOPMENTAL INTERVENTION WITH YOUNG PHYSICALLY HANDICAPPED CHILDREN

Developmental Intervention With Young Physically Handicapped Children

By

PHILIP L. SAFFORD, Ph.D.

Associate Professor Special Education
Kent State University, Kent, Ohio

and

DENA C. ARBITMAN, M.A.

Nursery School Supervisor
Cleveland Society for Crippled Children
Cleveland, Ohio

With a Foreword by

William B. Townsend, M.A.

Executive Director, Cleveland Society for Crippled Children
Cleveland, Ohio

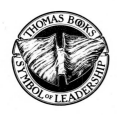

CHARLES C THOMAS · PUBLISHER
Springfield · Illinois · U.S.A.

Published and Distributed Throughout the World by
CHARLES C THOMAS · PUBLISHER
Bannerstone House
301-327 East Lawrence Avenue, Springfield, Illinois, U.S.A.

© *1975, by* CHARLES C THOMAS · PUBLISHER
ISBN 0-398-03326-9
Library of Congress Catalog Card Number: 75-7821

*With THOMAS BOOKS careful attention is given to all details of
manufacturing and design. It is the Publisher's desire to present books that are
satisfactory as to their physical qualities and artistic possibilities and
appropriate for their particular use. THOMAS BOOKS will be true to those
laws of quality that assure a good name and good will.*

Printed in the United States of America
M-3

To William B. Townsend who, with his unyielding dedication, unrelenting optimism, and extraordinary vision, has immeasurably enhanced the lives of countless numbers of handicapped children.

FOREWORD

THE CLEVELAND SOCIETY for Crippled Children, founded in 1940, is primarily concerned with meeting basic rehabilitation needs of children and youth from infancy to twenty years of age who have an orthopedic or related handicap, and with serving their families. Before our Society came into being, surveys had focused attention upon both the gaps in and the fragmentation of essential patient services for the handicapped, in both the private and public sectors. We recognized the role of our agency as being a catalytic factor in examining the programs and structural development of existing services. By a process of studied implementation, we worked to create a public consciousness of these unmet needs and to develop the Society as a multi-service agency.

Throughout its thirty-four year history, the Cleveland Society for Crippled Children has directed its energies to assure every handicapped child the benefits of the great accomplishments in ongoing research in medicine, education, psychology, therapy, and social work. Realization of this objective has frequently required the implementation of pioneering efforts on the part of the Society. The dedicated volunteers who have served as members of the agency's Board of Trustees have consistently demonstrated the faith and sense of leadership necessary to encourage innovation and to establish and to work toward long-range goals.

In order to establish a multi-service, consonant agency with a philosophy of comprehensive service, a sound organizational framework and professional program were developed which brought together the various disciplines which are required to achieve maximum rehabilitation goals. It was recognized that each of these professions had within its framework of training and experience significant knowledge and skill which, if optimally integrated, would contribute toward the achievement of objectives of the interdisciplinary rehabilitation team.

During these years the Society has also devoted its energies toward the development of adequate facilities and now operates two rehabilitation centers and Camp Cheerful, a year-round residential health camp for handicapped children and youth. The Society also established the first preschool classes in Cleveland for handicapped youngsters. Through these classes, handicapped children from three to six years of age are afforded the opportunity of a unique program concerned with physical restoration as well as group life experience. Attention is also focused upon the personal-social adjustment and the intellectual growth of every child, in order to assist him in utilizing his full potential and to prepare him for entrance into regular or special school.

An experiential review of the history of the Cleveland Society for Crippled Children reflects growth and innovation in the delivery of a wide range of health care and educative services. Now the authors of this book, with insight and expertise, have assembled a body of information which will add a bright new chapter to this history.

The Cleveland Foundation, one of the first community trusts in the United States, agreed in January of 1972 to support for two years the Heman Early Education Development Project, referred to in this book as Project HEED. The Foundation allocated grants from the Constance C. Frackleton and the David C. Wright Memorial Funds to finance this undertaking. While early intervention has been a hallmark in all of the agency's treatment and day-care programs, we were abled through these grants to establish on a demonstration basis an intensive program designed to foster the development and learning of younger physically disabled children. These youngsters, ranging in age from eighteen through thirty-six months, have associated disabilities as well as physical handicapping conditions. In Project HEED, individualized habilitation and teaching are provided by a multidiscipline staff, with particular emphasis given to gross and fine motor functions, cognitive growth, and social-emotional development. Although parent involvement and participation characterize all of the Society's programs, in Project HEED the parent component is given particular emphasis. The various services incorporated in the operation of HEED include physical therapy, education, occupational therapy, speech pathology, parent counseling, psychological testing, and transportation. The strategies through which these services have been incorporated in the form of an integrated team approach are described in this book, as are the assessment procedures which have been developed by the HEED team.

The Cleveland Society for Crippled Children has endeavored to carry on over the years the responsibilities for helping infants, children and youth who have serious disabilities. Through their detailed documentation and thoughtful analyses of the many facets of a promising approach to early intervention, the authors of this text have striven to extend the impact of our efforts.

William B. Townsend, M.A.

PREFACE

THIS BOOK PROVIDES A comprehensive treatment of habilitative work with and teaching of young physically handicapped children. The vehicle employed for this purpose is a
detailed documentation and analysis of a unique interdisciplinary early intervention project for children between the ages of
eighteen months and three years who have serious physical
handicaps and associated disabilities, including mental retardation, language problems and special socio-emotional needs.

Following a discussion of the nature of specific handicapping
conditions in children and the contemporary social context for
work with these children and their families, a rationale for the
value of early intervention is developed which draws on
psychological theories of cognitive and personal-social development. Project HEED is then related to the broader context of fundamental issues, trends, and approaches of contemporary early childhood education.

The interdisciplinary team approach is described, with particular emphasis on communications across professional lines,
integrated as opposed to compartmentalized planning and direct service, and procedures for observing, recording, and
evaluating children's progress. Special consideration is given to
the essential role of parents and to ways parents and professional staff can work together to bring about maximum impact
of the habilitative program. The components of and the techniques employed in carrying out a group educational program
for very young children with special needs are described in
detail, together with their theoretical rationale. An important
feature of the group program is the integration of therapy and
teaching goals and techniques, based on recognition of the
interrelatedness of motor functioning, cognitive growth, and
personality development in young children. Certain of these
goals and techniques are incorporated in a practically-oriented

curriculum guide through which the theories of Jean Piaget are applied to the teaching and habilitation of very young developmentally impaired children.

Philip L. Safford
Dena C. Arbitman

ACKNOWLEDGMENTS

IT IS IMPOSSIBLE FOR US to think of Project HEED without experiencing deep admiration for our dedicated co-workers, whose expertise, energy, and, most of all, whose humanity breathed life into the program. Some members of the HEED team have contributed material directly to this book, and their contributions are in each case duly recognized. All, however, have contributed to this effort in a multitude of ways and have greatly enriched our own understanding. For these contributions and for their candid criticisms and steadfast support we are indebted to Charlotte Baum, Mary Lou Boynton, Marguerite Campbell, Laura Gregg, Carole Lasko, Patricia MacIntyre, Ann Newman, Cynthia Prufer, Glenda Schneider and Janice Sewell. The special appreciation due William B. Townsend has been expressed in the form of the dedication of this book.

Drs. Donald K. Freedheim and John Jacobs reviewed major portions of the manuscript and offered many helpful suggestions, both substantive and stylistic, as did Dr. John Makley concerning our handling of medical portions. We are particularly indebted to Emma Plank who provided, in addition to the inspiration of her self and her work, a critical reading of the manuscript. We are grateful to Judith Arbitman, who shared with us her insights as a pediatric nurse, and to Clarice Lengyel, who permitted us to draw heavily on her experience in medical casework. The expert guidance we were privileged to employ has added immeasurably to our understanding.

To Helena Mencl, who carried out the long and tedious task of typing the manuscript, and to Bonnie Baskin and Janet Hawkins for their assistance in typing innumerable drafts and revisions, we extend our deep appreciation. A special word of thanks is due Richard Zelman for his assistance in preparing the plan view of the HEED classroom, and to Helen Smith for her editorial assistance.

Detailed follow-up observations of many of the children involved in the program were supplied by nursery school teachers of the Society for Crippled Children. For their time and concern we owe a great deal to Kelly Croyle, Kim Einstein, Elaine Jessup, Jane Safford, Laurel Taichnar and Barbara Williams.

A grant from The Cleveland Foundation made it possible to establish and maintain Project HEED for the past two years. We are grateful for that support and sincerely hope that we have fulfilled our promises.

We owe an enormous debt to all the "HEED Kids" who served as a constant inspiration and to their parents for their unwavering confidence in us.

And finally, to our respective families for their encouragement, patience and forbearance during the many long months we spent writing and revising, we express a heartfelt and long overdue "Thank you."

Project HEED, and this book which it has generated, involved so many as participants, consultants, advisors, and supporters that we have contracted a multitude of debts. Our only hope of repayment is that the work in which we have engaged for the past two years will, in some measure, be of help to handicapped youngsters and their families as well as to those professionals whose lives are devoted to serving them.

CONTENTS

	Page
Foreword	vii
Preface	xi
Acknowledgments	xiii

Chapter

1. THE HANDICAPPED CHILD IN CONTEMPORARY SOCIETY 3
2. HANDICAPPING CONDITIONS AND PSYCHOLOGICAL
   DEVELOPMENT IN YOUNG CHILDREN 21
3. PROJECT HEED: PURPOSES AND RATIONALE
   CONTEXT OF THE PROJECT: CONTEMPORARY EARLY
   CHILDHOOD EDUCATION 39
4. THE FORMATIVE EVALUATION PROCESS 56
5. PARENTS AND THEIR HANDICAPPED CHILDREN 80
6. PARENTS IN THE PROGRAM: MODES OF HELPING 96
7. THE EARLY LEARNING ENVIRONMENT 114
8. INDIVIDUALIZED THERAPY IN THE GROUP SETTING 132
9. PROMOTING SELF-AWARENESS AND BODY MASTERY 149
10. PROMOTING PEER AWARENESS AND SOCIAL INTERACTION 164
11. PROMOTING COGNITIVE AND LANGUAGE LEARNING 181
12. CONSIDERATIONS AND APPROACHES IN BEHAVIOR
    MANAGEMENT 210
13. CASE STUDIES OF REPRESENTATIVE CHILDREN 226
14. EVALUATION OF PROJECT HEED: THE CHILDREN 249
15. CONCLUSIONS: THE IMPACT OF COMPREHENSIVE
    INTERVENTION 270

Bibliography 289
Appendix A: GOALS AND PROGRESS RECORD FORM 293
Appendix B: EDUCATION ASSESSMENT INSTRUMENTS 294
Appendix C: PHYSICAL THERAPY ASSESSMENT INSTRUMENTS 297
Appendix D: OCCUPATIONAL THERAPY ASSESSMENT INSTRUMENTS 303

xv

Appendix E: CASEWORK ASSESSMENT INSTRUMENT 307
Appendix F: HEED PARENT QUESTIONNAIRE 311
Appendix G: PLAN VIEW OF HEED CLASSROOM 313
Index 315

DEVELOPMENTAL INTERVENTION
WITH YOUNG
PHYSICALLY HANDICAPPED CHILDREN

CHAPTER 1

THE HANDICAPPED CHILD IN CONTEMPORARY SOCIETY

YESTERDAY AND TODAY

ATTITUDES TOWARD PHYSICAL disabilities reflect a composite of religious ideology, early myths, superstitions, and modern day scientific knowledge.

From the earliest days of recorded history human beings have been afflicted with physical abnormalities. Egyptian and Babylonian tablets and sculptures depict individuals with limbs missing, cleft lips and various other abnormalities. The Bible reports that King Saul's son Ishboshet was born crippled. Achondroplastic dwarfs served as court jesters to Roman emperors. Because ancient peoples sought to understand the reason for such afflictions but lacked specific information, superstitions arose. Responsibility rested on the affected individual who was often shunned, feared and left to die or on the family who was viewed as suffering the act of a vengeful god for past misdeeds. As religious views were imposed upon pagan rites and practices, Judaism wrestled with the ethical problem of why the righteous suffer; Job's sorry plight was explained as a testing of his faith and not a punishment. Christianity viewed suffering as purifying and ennobling, a means of attaining grace.

Although modern research has given us the scientific and naturalistic answers for the causes of many physical malformations, even today there is widespread acceptance of the belief that physical differences, even within a normal range of variation, are indicators of personality and character traits. The man with wide-spaced eyes is popularly assumed to possess greater integrity than one whose eyes are small and set close together. The person possessing a stout, well-rounded body is believed to be more jovial and generous than his lean counterpart. Police departments, recently under fire for hiring policies which discriminate against certain minority groups, have defended their height requirements as an eligibility factor for employment by insisting that tall officers inspire greater respect for authority than short ones.

If physical differences that fall within the accepted normal range elicit such definite reactions, then it is not surprising that the dwarf, the spina bifida, and the amputee induce even more potent emotional responses.

Perhaps the fears which were incorporated in ancient superstitions still lurk in the corners of more enlightened minds. The cripple was once believed invested with a supernatural power to perform evil and was therefore to be avoided as dangerous. The belief that he is suffering the consequences of a moral transgression and therefore *bad* may still be a factor responsible for avoidance by others. Or perhaps on an unconscious level there is a projection of one's own fears which supports the belief that the handicapped are dangerous.

Within the past decade, the need to improve all aspects of human relations, i.e. people's ability to accept other people, has received great attention. Legislation has been enacted to protect the rights of minority groups and widely held myths have been attacked. Racial and ethnic stereotypes are no longer considered fitting subjects for humor. Yet television, movies and newspaper comics still reflect and perhaps reinforce general attitudes about physical malformation by creating characters with bulbous noses, missing legs, awkward gaits, speech disorders, hearing impairments, strabismus and dwarfism as a way of depicting horror or comedy. Society's attitudes toward the physically handicapped need to be reviewed and revised in order to dispel myths. A child with celebral palsy who lurches when he walks is not evil or monstrous but a child whose muscular activity has been impaired by damage to his brain. Midgets and dwarfs are not comic characters or buffoons but usually people of normal intelligence whose stature is a result of a genetic disorder.

As explanations of birth anomalies based on scientific data are more widely disseminated by means of newspaper and

Cerebral palsy is characterized by weakness, paralysis and an inability to control muscle reflexes. Marcus, a child with mild involvement, seems awkward and clumsy, unable to "walk and chew gum simultaneously." His lack of coordination extends to poor hand coordination and sloppy eating habits. Julia, a severely involved child, is unable to sit unaided, speaks unintelligibly and requires almost total physical care. Most children with cerebral palsy fall somewhere between those two extremes.

Cerebral palsy, a static condition, one which cannot be cured but is by definition not progressive (Keats, 1973), is often divided into three groups: spasticity, athetosis, and ataxia. The child who is spastic may be very rigid; the legs scissor and increased activity of deep tendon reflexes often cause contractures. Despite the fact that the disorder is not progressive, the dual factors of growth and spasticity may contribute to the development of further deformities. For spastic children, therefore, growth may create a dynamic and evolving problem requiring careful orthopedic supervision. The child with athetosis makes many involuntary movements. Julia knew where to place the pieces of the formboard, but her arm movements were so uncontrolled and explosive that she frequently swept the entire puzzle off the table. The ataxic lacks balance and depth perception. There is a high incidence of mental retardation as well as perceptual and speech disorders in cerebral palsied children (Telford and Sawrey, 1972).

One can speculate that because cerebral palsied children seem to expend such great energy in making their muscles obey their bidding, many of them tend to become lethargic and unmotivated to explore their environment or to participate in activities. They require physical therapy to keep from developing contractures and pressure sores and stimulation to keep them interested in activities appropriate to their age and development.

Myelodysplasia

Myelodysplasia, or spina bifida, occurs in approximately three of every 1,000 babies (Nelson, Vaughan & McKay,

1969). It is an abnormality of the spinal cord which occurs when one or more of the vertebrae are not completely formed. In a mild form a dimple or a tuft of hair is noted, but in more severe forms a sac, a myelomeningocele, protrudes at the point of the lesion and is filled with fluid, spinal nerve roots and malformed cord. The legs and trunk below the lesion are usually paralyzed and frequently bladder and bowel control are impossible. Often the myelomeningocele is removed shortly after birth, but it is impossible to restore function to the lower trunk and legs. Children with myelodysplasia often have hydrocephalus; they are prone to kidney and bladder infections and pressure sores, as well as bone deformities such as dislocated hips.

Many children with myelodysplasia learn to walk with long leg braces and crutches. Many hours of physical therapy and skill and patience on the part of the therapist are required, for many of these children cannot feel the floor with the soles of their feet. The belief is often expressed by those who work with such children, therefore, that because of their lack of sensation in the lower extremities, they must indeed take the therapist's word on pure faith when they first venture forth on crutches.

Hydrocephalus

This condition has sometimes been referred to by the layman as "water on the brain." It is caused by retention of intracranial fluid around the brain because an obstruction keeps the fluid from reaching a point from which absorption can take place. The incidence of hydrocephalus is three per one thousand births. The condition is usually identified within the first few weeks after birth and treatment usually consists of bypassing the obstruction by shunting the cerebrospinal fluid by means of a plastic tube which is inserted surgically into a ventricle. Hydrocephalus, when untreated, often causes an increase in head size and pressure on the brain. Unless a spontaneous remission occurs or there is medical intervention, death usually ensues. Although use of the shunt is widely accepted, difficulties can occur because of infections, blockage and the need for shunt revisions. However, the shunting process, when performed early in infancy, has enabled many children to lead more satisfying lives.

Clubfoot

The condition known as clubfoot is characterized by a foot which is generally twisted inward and bent so that the heel is in an upward position and the ankle and outside edge of the foot touch the floor. The incidence is one in three hundred babies, and until recently it was believed that the baby's position in the uterus caused the malformation. However, this theory is no longer considered valid. The condition requires orthopedic treatment by means either of a plaster cast or bandaging and a splint in conjunction with manipulation and stretching. A metal bar attached to corrective shoes is sometimes prescribed to hold the feet in the correct position while the child is sleeping. When conservative treatment of this form is not effective, surgery is performed. Although sometimes after the deformity has been corrected there is a recurrence, early treatment and regular check-ups generally permit the child to lead a normal life.

Congenital or Surgical Amputee

The child amputee may have been born with congenital absence of an arm or leg or the limb may have been surgically removed because it was vestigial and nonfunctional or because of injury or malignancy. In any case the child who is fitted for a prosthesis early adjusts to its use more easily. Very young children can be taught to walk with a reasonably good gait if they have a properly fitted prosthesis. Physical therapists can help by checking on the condition of the stump and by providing gait training insuring a proper fit of the prosthesis. Successful use of the prosthesis depends on the family's encouragement of its use. Teachers also need to understand the mechanics of the artificial limb, particularly if it is an arm prosthesis, and they should be prepared to present activities which require its use to accomplish the tasks. The amputee whose family, therapist, and teacher help him develop confidence in himself can live a full and productive life.

Phocomelia

Phocomelia is a deformity of the extremities. The portion of the limb closest to the body is reduced in size so that the end of the limb (hands or feet) is near the trunk. For example, in complete phocomelia the hand or foot seems to be directly attached to the trunk of the body.

Osteogenesis Imperfecta

Osteogenesis imperfecta is a congenital disorder characterized by fragile bones which fracture easily. Because fractures may occur before birth and heal in abnormal positions, the infant is often born with deformities. Fractures generally heal satisfactorily but are replaced by inferior bone so that further deformities develop. Although bone age corresponds to chronological age, in the continuing process of fracturing and healing, the bones assume grotesque shapes and the individual's growth is usually stunted. In the most severe form of the disease the chest and spine are deformed. In its milder form, osteogenesis imperfecta tarda, fractures are less frequent and fragility of the bones ceases with puberty.

Arthrogryposis

Arthrogryposis is a congenital stiffness of the joints along with defective development of muscle tissue. There is an inward rotation of the arms, and an outward rotation of the thighs; club feet are usually present. The wrists and fingers are flexed and dimples often appear in the skin at the joints. In severe cases the child may be confined to a wheelchair; in less severe cases bracing, orthopedic surgery, and intensive physical therapy may be helpful in facilitating ambulation.

Juvenile Rheumatoid Arthritis

Exact figures on incidence are not available, but the disease is not rare. Although the cause is unknown, onset often follows injury or infection. It is characterized by inflammation of the affected joints, and tendon and muscle inflammation may also occur. The affected joint becomes swollen and tender to touch and movement. In the morning, after naps or similar periods of inactivity, the child may suffer stiffness which inhibits his ability to rise quickly from bed or chair. Children with rheumatoid arthritis may suffer periods of irritability and loss of appetite.

Although there is no known cure, the disease is not life-threatening and the chances for remission are good. The child should not be over-indulged and permitted to become an invalid. Children who have rheumatoid arthritis should be encouraged to care for their own needs and to lead full lives.

Achondroplastic Dwarfism

Achondroplasia is a disorder affecting the cartilage. Because the long bones are most affected, as the child grows the body becomes disproportioned and dwarfism results. The achondroplastic dwarf has a normal trunk, shortened and curved extremities, large head and protruding buttocks. The pelvis is often deformed and this produces a waddling gait.

This condition begins before birth, and genetic factors are involved. Children with achondroplasia usually enjoy good health and are of normal intelligence. There is no specific treatment except orthopedic correction of deformities as they develop to improve appearance and physical therapy to aid in ambulation.

Legg-Calvé Perthes Disease

In Perthes disease the head of the femur which fits into the socket formed by the hip becomes diseased. For unknown reasons the tissues at the head of the femur begin to die. This occurs more frequently in males than females, and usually the age at onset is between four and ten years. The child begins to limp and complains of pain in the hip and knee.

While the process involving the tissue death is going on, weight must be kept off the involved leg or the head of the femur tends to become flattened and mushroom shaped. Untreated, this would cause later degenerative changes because the head of the femur would no longer fit properly into the acetabulum (socket) of the hip.

Treatment once involved complete bed rest with traction on the legs. More recently, however, orthopedists immobilize the hip using casts or braces to remove weight, but allow the child some freedom of movement. The younger the child is at onset, the better his chances of avoiding flattening of the head of the femur. Complete recovery depends upon severity of the deformity and promptness of treatment.

Bowleg and Knock-Knees

Bowleg and knock-knees are considered developmental variants which are usually corrected by growth. When the ligaments of the knees stretch, however, braces are not employed as a correction for the deformity but as a prevention of further stretching of the ligaments. Bowleg, which results from a tibial deformity, Blounts disease, may also require bracing. Children who have already experienced independent ambulation often exhibit anger at the restraint imposed by long leg braces and need opportunities to express their feelings.

ILLNESS AND ACCIDENT

Sometimes an illness which occurs in infancy or early childhood leaves residual effects which necessitate medical and rehabilitative services for years to come. High fevers of unknown origin, meningitis, encephalitis and sometimes unidentified viral infections can cause cerebral damage. Complications of meningitis, for example, include nervous system disorders, paralysis and spasticity. The symptoms of a child whose brain damage results from illness may be very similar to the symptoms of a child suffering from a birth defect.

Automobile accidents, falls from heights and poison ingestion all take their toll during the early years.

Although the nursery school enrollments in rehabilitative agencies typically reflect a relatively small percentage of children who have suffered trauma due to injury or illness, those children and their families require the same supportive services as the ones affected by birth defects. In fact, families often require more intensive counseling to enable them to understand the changes in the child, depending on age at onset of the disability, and the child may need help in expressing the anger and frustration which often arise when the body is no longer as responsive as it once was.

SERVICES

Medical treatment, rehabilitation, education and institutionalization all require huge outlays of money from the family, the state and federal governments, and voluntary philanthropic organizations. The financial resources of individual families are rarely adequate to cover the costly long-term treatment required for the maintenance of a physically handicapped child, but government subsidies are often available through State Bureau for the Handicapped. School districts receive varying amounts of extra compensation from state tax revenues for the education of exceptional children in special classes, in hospitals, and at home. In an attempt to discover answers concerning cause, prevention and amelioration of specific diseases, a number of organizations have engaged in exhaustive research as well as in the dissemination of accurate scientific information to families involved and to the general public. The National Foundation/March of Dimes is just one of the numerous organizations which have made noteworthy contributions in this area.

Aside from the considerable financial responsibility, there is a need for diverse professional expertise. Many communities have established clinics, often hospital based, which offer the services of teams of physicians in the fields of pediatrics, orthopedics and neurology, and those of clinical psychologists, caseworkers, educators and physical, occupational, and speech therapists who supply supportive and rehabilitative help to child and family.

The needs of parents for authoritative and practical guides to caring for their physically handicapped child has been addressed by individuals of such eminence as Benjamin Spock (Spock and Lerrigo, 1965) and Virginia Apgar (Apgar and Beck, 1972). The mechanical aspects of facilitating movement, positions, and relieving spastic muscles in children with cerebral palsy have been effectively communicated through pictorial representation in a book by Nancie Finnie (1970).

Although increasing numbers of exceptional children are being cared for in their own homes, residential institutions must be maintained for those who require them. State supported residential schools vary considerably in quality, but recent trends have been in the direction of upgrading personnel and educational services. Wherever possible, handicapped children are being educated in their own communities, and families are encouraged through financial assistance and supportive services to keep the children at home. However, it is sometimes impossible for the family to provide the care necessary for a severely handicapped youngster. Where this is the case, such children should be assured proper care and an appropriate educational program in a residential school.

Where nursery school programs are not available through local school districts, agencies such as The Society for Crippled Children operate nursery schools for children with on-going medical problems. These programs provide early intervention and modifications and adaptations of equipment and curricula in an attempt to ameliorate and, whenever possible, prevent the secondary impairments which may arise from lack of mobility or lack of exposure to peers and to equipment or materials appropriate to the three to five-year-old in his cognitive, emotional, and social development.

SPECIAL EDUCATION PROGRAMS

Communities usually provide classes which are equipped to serve the needs of exceptional children. To facilitate operation several districts often combine to maintain one school building or a complex of buildings which serves as a center for children with a variety of handicapping conditions. Children with visual and hearing impairments, orthopedic handicaps and neurological disorders are transported to one location which provides physical plant, trained teachers, therapy and educational equipment appropriate to their needs.

Therapists based in one building can provide more units of service each day than is possible if travel is added to their schedule. This kind of setting permits a more reasonable cost in the purchase and maintenance of the facility and its special equipment and offers convenience in the supervision of teachers and the administration of programs. Curriculum can be planned and implemented for special needs and the child-teacher ratio maintained at a level which is advantageous to the child who requires more adult attention. Within a special setting handicapped youngsters, although basically a heterogeneous group, are less different from peers than they would be in regular schools and parents of exceptional children frequently feel more comfortable when their children are in a sheltered environment.

Long recognized as an important area of special education, the topic of educational services and programming for the physically handicapped has been addressed by many leaders in the field. (See, for example, Cruickshank and Johnson, 1967.)

Despite current sociological and political trends in the United States which seek to minimize differences, exceptional children do have needs which are different from those of other children in the community. To ignore this basic fact does not obliterate the needs but may give rise to inadequate or inappropriate planning.

EXCEPTIONAL CHILDREN IN REGULAR CLASSROOMS

Many exceptional children attend regular classes not because of educational and social philosophy but because there are no special centers available. Teachers in regular classrooms are familiar with the child who requires attention in either greater measure or in different ways than the majority of their pupils. How successfully teachers have coped with the situation depends on the individual teacher's skills and attitudes and the student's ability and motivation to utilize them.

Recent trends have encouraged, or as in the case of Head Start, mandated, the integration of handicapped children into regular classes. Although the sudden implementation of such programming may be overwhelming to teachers and administrators, often the problems encountered are less catastrophic than anticipated.

The emotional reaction to braces and crutches or to a wheelchair or a prosthetic limb may be so overwhelming to those who have had no experience with handicapped children that the initial response may be to the applicance and not to the child. In their consternation and embarrassment teachers and principals may cite the lack of proper physical facilities as a reason for exclusion of the child. Architectural barriers are a poor excuse for excluding a child from the education to which he is entitled, and parents, therapists, or social workers can often help school personnel to make the adjustments necessary to accommodate the handicapped child. Sometimes, for example, all that is required is the addition of a hand rail in the lavatory or that the child be excused five minutes earlier or later than the rest of the class. Fortunately, as planners of new public buildings are made aware of the needs of the handicapped, architectural accommodations, such as ramps, wider doorways, hand rails, and elevators are being incorporated to aid not only the orthopedically handicapped, but the elderly, as well as those suffering from cardiac and other chronic medical conditions.

An understanding of the child's disability and of the treatment involved often helps dispel the initial fear caused by visual impact of the appliance. Fortunately, exceptional children also possess many normal traits which make them not totally unlike other children and, as teachers begin to understand this through association with handicapped children, their anxieties abate.

If children with handicaps are to remain within their communities as productive members of society, then accepting them into regular schools is imperative for it is through experiences with non-handicapped peers that they will learn to function effectively in the mainstream.

ALTERNATIVE APPROACHES

Within the general field of special education, the range of options available for accommodating the exceptional child within the education system has been significantly expanded in recent years. A variety of strategies and programs have been proposed for adoption, depending upon the *educational* needs of the individual child (Deno, 1973).

There are several alternatives for accomplishing the integration of exceptional children in regular educational settings:

(1) Integration of all children regardless of physical, mental or emotional problems into regular classrooms. All teachers would need to be trained to work with all children or teachers trained in special education would have to be available on a prescriptive basis.

(2) Integration of only those children whose physical disability does not hinder their functioning effectively in a regular classroom. A therapy program prescribed for individual needs would be available, preferably at the school or at a central location to which the child would be transported during released time.

(3) Partial integration by means of special classes held in

regular schools. This would permit children to attend the same school as siblings and playmates and would remove the stigma attached to attendance at a special school. Contact with peers would not be interrupted by the need for travel to a distant location which removes the child from the neighborhood for many hours each day over the span of his school years. Because special and regular classes would be held on the same site, two benefits would accrue: (a) integrated activities could be planned when appropriate, and (b) integration of a child who is ready for the regular program could be accomplished gradually by lengthening his stay in the regular classroom, thus minimizing the effects of the transition.

The availability of educators and therapists trained to work with exceptional children would enrich the expertise of all the teachers and the non-handicapped students would benefit from continuing experience with handicapped children.

The nursery school in a special setting might serve as a means of providing intensive therapies and training in activities of daily living and self-care, i.e. ambulation, toileting, and feeding. This early experience could provide the child with a foundation for developing social and cognitive skills, becoming able to separate from home, and learning to follow school routines. At an even earlier age a program similar to Project HEED, described in subsequent chapters of this book, could provide sensory stimulation and intensive therapy to the child as well as serve the parent. Thus, within a short time after identification, rehabilitative and educational intervention would begin to prepare the child to enter the mainstream of life as quickly as possible.

Chapters 2,3, and 4 present the rationale and foundation for an interdisciplinary team approach to early intervention for young handicapped children and their families. The approach itself, together with its ramifications for those who work with such children, is the subject of the discussion in the remaining chapters.

CHAPTER **2**

HANDICAPPING CONDITIONS AND PSYCHOLOGICAL DEVELOPMENT IN YOUNG CHILDREN

INTERACTIVE PROCESSES OF DEVELOPMENT

ALTHOUGH IT IS POSSIBLE on an intellectual level to consider human development as comprising parallel streams —mental, physical, and socio-emotional—these areas are, in practice, reciprocally related and perhaps inseparable. Just as cognition and affect interact, so do psyche and soma. Traditionally, specialists in therapeutic education and rehabilitation have given at least lip service to the relationship by observing, for example, that an orthopedically handicapped individual will certainly have feelings about himself relating to his physical problem and that his handicap will in some measure color his relationship with his social environment. Consequently, while attempting to enable the individual to maximize his competencies, rehabilitation efforts hopefully give due emphasis to his self-feelings, relative to his sense of competence and self-worth, his psychological need to function as independently as possible, and his ability to deal with the responses of nonhandicapped individuals to his problem.

The relation between mind and body is, however, undoubtedly much more subtle and complex than this. Since Descartes, few serious thinkers would maintain that these are separate entities. The implication would appear to be that it is not enough to guide the individual toward a mental state which allows him to adjust to a physical limitation. A person cannot be considered independently of his physical being, for we do not thus view ourselves. Psychological theorists with special concern

21

for the exceptional individual, such as Newell Kephart, have insisted on the centrality of motor activity in the genesis of intellect. Current interest in body language, or nonverbal communication, and the Gestalt school of psychotherapy give further credence to the continuing unity throughout life of body and mind.

Developmental theorists, such as Jean Piaget, note that mental structures evolve from sensorimotor roots, that cognitive modes such as hypothetico-deductive thinking evolve from foundations laid in earliest infancy. To Piaget, thought is an active process, a principle which is true in the literal sense of overt, physical acts during the first two years of life.

FROM DEPENDENCE TO INDEPENDENCE

During the early years, learning occurs at a fantastic pace, relative to the rate at which our capabilities are subsequently modified. Compared to many other species, of course, humans become capable of independent activity and self-sufficiency much more slowly.

Most children, however, by the time they have reached age four, have already mastered a great many of the most important tasks they will ever undertake. The most fundamental of these, those with the widest ramifications of influence in virtually all spheres of development, are learning to move about and ultimately to stand erect and walk, and learning to use language as a communicative and information processing system.

The experiential world of the newborn infant is a rather limited one. Although visual focusing and tracking have been observed in infants during the first few days of life (Kessen, 1967; Fantz and Nevis, 1967), the visual world of the infant is very restricted indeed. It may be that the observed capability to track objects, together with pronounced preferences for certain visual forms, provides a motivational impetus to the baby to alter his body position and to become mobile. Pronounced differences in the activities of children who can attain a sitting position from their earlier modes of environmental exploration suggest how this achievement of a new physical orientation capability can affect play behavior, manipulation of objects, and processing of new sensory impressions. This change of the experienced environment from a lie-down to a sit-up world must have profound implications for the development of thought.

Similarly, the ability to move about and the accompanying urge to explore the environment, observed so commonly by parents of pre-ambulatory children, changes radically what the child is able to experience. His psychological environment is broadened so rapidly that fearful parents are often disposed to intervene as a "creeper" makes straight for an electrical outlet, a door, or the family dog.

Standing erect, aided for a time by a low table or chair arm, brings new capabilities for experiencing the environment. And walking is the crowning achievement! The first step toward a parent's outstretched hands is an unparalleled triumph.

The second major achievement, the acquisition of language, similarly has its roots in very early spontaneous behavior; the babbling of infancy, in an amazingly short period of time, becomes communicative speech. When one considers how laborious the process of learning to read is for so many learners, it becomes still more surprising that the ability is acquired with such little apparent effort on the part of the child or conscious teaching on the part of adults to understand and to use accurately and creatively a spoken language system.

While still a preschooler, a child has learned that, in addition to their social significance, words and word sequences have an important function of *representing* (not being identical with) things, people, places, actions and even abstract ideas, such as love, which he regularly experiences. This awareness of the distinction between the symbol and that which it represents (the object itself) provides him with a source of enormous new power. He now has a system for representing internally the complexities of the objective environment, thus rendering them subjectively meaningful.

If during the first year or so of life a child is able to gain a sense that the world is basically benign and that he is valued and will be cared for, a sense which Erik Erikson (1950) has termed *basic trust*, he is better equipped to begin to establish himself as an individual in his own right. He can become a person, aware of himself as a separate entity, and aware of his own power to alter both his physical and social environment. Valued and loved by important others, he must become competent in terms of control of his own body and those events which impinge upon him. The classic scenario for this, as the psychoanalytic writers have frequently observed, is the drama surrounding toilet training. The crisis is more generalized than merely the gain of sphincter control, however, as Erikson has conveyed through his concept of the developmental conflict relating to *Autonomy* vs. *Shame* and *Doubt*. For the toddler, establishing himself as a person aware of himself and his own competence is often marked by declarations of independence, and the code word for these is "No!"

Difficult as these times may be for parents of "the terrible two's," the assertion of selfhood, of potency, even for a time, fantasies of omnipotence, are recognized as important developmental milestones. Bruno Bettleheim (1967) has observed in older autistic children the absence of assertions of ownership or self-identification. A psychological experience of efficacy, to use Robert White's (1959) term, appears a highly motivating condition for learning in relation to both the social and physical environment. Not negating the traditional view that human young, like other species, respond to environmental stimuli which impinge upon them, the idea of effectance motivation posits that the ability of the child to influence his environment, that is, to be able to affect or to alter it through his own actions, is intrinsically motivating. The more success a child has in effecting change, the more likely he will be to continue in such attempts.

In all such transactions with objects during the first two years of life, reception and expression capabilities go hand in hand. At first, movement itself appears to be gratifying and self-sustaining. What Buhler (1930) termed *function pleasure* is reflected in the use of limbs, attempts to shift position, to turn the head. Reflex patterns, such as the startle response and the rooting reflex, can be said to reflect innate adaptive mechanisms. Although these reflexes disappear, others come to be used with increasing selectivity and to be increasingly differentiated with cumulative experience and constant refinement of coordination. Movements become increasingly intentional and goal-oriented.

The acquisition of language capabilities for receiving, processing, and conveying information is certainly related to thought and feeling. However, the nature of the developmental relationships involved is by no means thoroughly resolved, nor is the issue of precisely what processes account for the origins of speech. That the congenitally deaf, who have never heard spoken language, suffer an enormous handicap with respect to subsequent acquisition of both a communicative mode and cognitive learning goes without saying. However, the investigations of Hans Furth (1964) demonstrating conceptual capabilities among deaf children when a response means not requiring language is possible, would appear to support the position of Piaget (1969) that thought and language are independent processes.

FROM REFLEX TO SCHEMA

Thus, during the first two years of life the foundations of thinking are laid. Thought-as-action is established as the prototype of human intelligence. In Piaget's theory, the schemas which are formed are action patterns—internalizations of overt acts. They are the product of the infant's attempts to organize events and sensations involving his own body in relation to the physical environment with which he has contact.

Initially, he is not aware of the existence of objects as independent entities, not knowing where he leaves off and his environment begins. Establishment of the concept of the permanent object is a major accomplishment of this period of life. "The conquest of the object," as David Elkind (1970) has called it, is a necessary precursor to concepts *about* objects and their spatial relationships and attributes, i.e. to conceptualization itself.

The importance of concepts in mental development has been increasingly stressed by theorists and empirical researchers in child development. In the words of Irving Sigel, one of the foremost researchers on children's thinking, concepts ". . . are the intellectual tools that man uses in organizing his environment and attacking his problems" (1964).

Piaget's descriptions of the emergence and coordination of sensorimotor schemas appear to assume the interaction of an intact organism with an adequate environment. In replications of Piaget's experiments and attempts to test his theories, researchers have frequently focused on environmental variations, that is, they have investigated the effects of impoverished or enriched environments on quantitative and qualitative aspects of cognitive growth. That organism characteristics may influence in important ways the form this necessary child-environment interaction may take has also been of interest to some investigators. However, with important exceptions, some of which will be discussed presently, these investigations have, for the most part, been restricted to comparisons of the functioning of mentally retarded with nonretarded individuals.

In analyzing Piaget's detailed and fascinating reports of his observations concerning early sensorimotor development within the context of his broader epistemological perspective, one might question how the absence of a limb, for example, or a partial paralysis, or difficulties effecting voluntary control of motor functions might affect the development of thought. According to Piaget, the infant is born with congenitally organized reflex capabilities, such as sucking and looking. Through a succession of increasingly complex elaborations and coordinations of motor acts and sensory feedback, called *circular reactions*, the infant acquires the ability to carry out intentionally a sequence such as the following: *Seeing* an object, he may *reach* for it, *grasp* it, *bring* it *toward him*, and *suck* on it. This sequence, observed commonly by parents, will be repeated with many objects and, at times, varied. Through such coordinated activities, the infant is taking in information about his world and about himself, information which is then applied to new situations.

Observation 137—At 0;8 (29) Laurent examines at length a notebook which he has just grasped. He transfers it from one hand to the other while turning it in all directions, touches the cover, then one of the corners, then the cover again, and finally the edge. Afterward he shakes himself, shakes his head while looking at it, displaces it more slowly with a wide motion and ends by rubbing it against the side of the bassinet. He then observes that in rubbing against the wicker the notebook does not produce the usual effect (sound? consistency?) and examines the contact most attentively while rubbing more gently (Piaget, 1952).

It seems apparent that a normally functioning organism is assumed in Piaget's formulations. The looking schema presupposes vision. Sucking presupposes function of various muscles in a coordinated fashion. Reaching is dependent upon flexor and extensor capabilities. Grasping requires prehension, which may initially be a far cry from the finely controlled finger-thumb teamwork which may in large measure account for man's evolutionary success story.

To Piaget, thought is based on physical actions performed in sequence, ultimately in order to achieve goals. Thus, what may begin as random motor activity rapidly becomes channeled in the service of the infant's mind. Not only are sequences which bring pleasure repeated, they are expanded and adapted in response to new environmental conditions. A change in the situation elicits invention (to use Piaget's term) of new strategies.

Another of Piaget's observations of one of his own children illustrates how problem solving is made possible by the child's motoric capabilities:

Observation 167—At 1;3 (12) Jacqueline throws a plush dog outside the bars of her playpen and she tries to catch it. Not succeeding, she then pushes the pen itself in the right direction! By holding onto the frame with one hand while with the other she tried to grasp the dog, she observed that the frame was mobile. She had accordingly, without wishing to do so, moved it away from the dog. She at once tried to correct this movement and thus saw the pen approach its objective. These two fortuitous discoveries then led her to utilize movements of the playpen and to push it at first experimentally, then systematically. There was a moment's groping, but it was short.

At 1;3 (16), on the other hand, Jacqueline right away pushes her playpen in the direction of the objects to be picked up. (Piaget, 1952).

ORIGINS OF THE SELF

When in the course of early development does a child become aware of himself as a person? When does he acquire the ability to be conscious of his own existence as a separate being from his experienced environment?

The first self-concept is a body image, a sense of one's physical existence, together with awareness of sensations, such as pain. Through the development of the concept of the independent object and the early formation of what H. S. Sullivan (1953) termed the *me-not-me* dichotomy, the child acquires awareness of his own body boundaries, where his own body parts end and that which is not his body begins. However, this learning requires the ability to gain necessary information through the senses and through the increasing ability to coordinate these sensory messages.

In terms of cognitive learning, the concept of self in a real sense underlies all other concepts. Learning about objects, for example, is accomplished through the child's own actions upon them and the feedback he receives. He does not initially distinguish between the action and the object; it is only through such transactions that a discrimination of self, the self-awareness so basic and essential to humanness, can be accomplished. As Piaget has described the course of cognitive development, the young child must essentially construct a universe, with himself at its center. In order to comprehend the notion of a "perspective," or "point of view," that is, to know that a situation might conceivably appear differently to another than it does to him simply because they view it from different angles and thus see different phenomena or relationships, he must accomplish what has often been called "a miniature Copernican revolution."

Self-evaluation in a very young child is probably inextricably interwoven both with self-awareness and feelings of effectiveness. Messages from important others in the social environment, in addition to the child's own actions on the physical environment, must certainly contribute greatly to this evaluative aspect of the self-concept. To affirm that a physically handicapped child, both during infancy and subsequently, has the same needs as any other child for love and esteem, for "unconditional positive regard" (Rogers, 1959), is certainly unnecessary. It would seem likely that, in many instances, the magnitude of these needs for assurance of love, safety, and security would be exacerbated by conditions associated with a physical problem, frequent or prolonged hospitalization, for example. Possibly the condition itself might endanger the growth of self. If oral feeling is impeded, one might fear for the development of basic trust.

EFFECTS OF EXPERIENTIAL DEPRIVATION

It has frequently been observed that parents of infants are assumed to provide stimulation of the six sensory modes, albeit on an unplanned and unsystematic basis, almost inevitably in the course of interaction which focuses mainly on affectional and caretaking activities. The desirability of visual, auditory, tactile, olfactory, gustatory, and kinesthetic stimulation for infants is recognized by parents almost intuitively, and in the normal course of events, these perceptive modes are exercised through provision of bright colors, fascinating sounds, and a constant variety of sensory impressions. The assumption is usually made that the infant whose receptors and central nervous system functioning are intact, given adequate environment, will acquire the necessary amount of appropriately paced experience to ensure normal perceptual and cognitive maturation.

Studies with institutionalized infants or those experiencing "deprived" early environmental conditions from the standpoint of perceptual and motor experience, such as the research of Dennis and Najarian (1957), have pointed to the importance of at least minimal quantities of stimulation in the environment.

The maternal deprivation hypothesis associated with the research of René Spitz (1945), as an explanatory factor for observed physical, mental and emotional anomalous development
and even mortality among infants in institutional settings has to
some extent given way to a sensory, experiential deprivation
hypothesis (Casler, 1965; Pinneau, 1950).

With respect to the effects on early sensorimotor development of severely visually handicapped or congenitally blind
children, Selma Fraiberg (1966) and her co-workers have presented evidence of apparent compensation. These children
demonstrate evidence of acquisition of the concept of the permanent object despite a handicapping condition which one
might presume would render impossible this necessary step
toward cognition. As Peter Wolff (1966) has observed, much
has yet to be learned concerning ways in which blind children
acquire such pivotal learnings necessary to the genesis of logical
thought as concepts of concrete physical space and orientation
of one's own body in space.

Regarding the interplay of tactile, kinesthetic and visual experiences, and the assumed intact physical organism alluded to
earlier, Wolff also cites preliminary findings obtained by
Gouin-Descaries (cited in Wolff, 1966) documenting acquisition of object permanence in thalidomide babies. Those infants
with hands but not arms, a condition preventing manipulation
of objects in front of the body and in the frontal visual field,
appear able nonetheless to master the concept of the permanent object.

Again, it is assumed that, optimally, hand and eye work
together from earliest tactile-visual explorations of objects.
Where interfering conditions exist with respect to visual function, arm and/or hand bone or muscle integrity, central nervous system functioning affecting the operation of either perceptive mode involved (visual, tactile, kinesthetic) or the voluntary coordination of these systems and processes, a number of
unresolved issues remain. What are the effects of such conditions, if any, on intellective development? What compensatory
processes may operate, if any, and how? Would external intervention serve to mitigate the effects of such a condition on

cognitive and general development? What form, or forms, should such intervention take? Are there critical periods in early development for intervention or particular kinds appropriate to handicapping conditions of particular kinds or should the rule for intervention be "the earlier the better, the more comprehensive the better?"

It would appear necessary at the very least to specify particular types or forms of handicap when attempting to consider the preceding questions. As was pointed out in Chapter 1, however, precise identification of types of handicapping conditions may at times be difficult. For one thing, various typologies have been applied to a general handicap classification, such as cerebral palsy. One may specify the type (spastic, athetoid, ataxic), number of limbs involved, degree of physical involvement, time of onset of the condition (prenatal, perinatal, postnatal), extent and nature of associated brain damage, related factors, such as measured intellectual level of functioning and psychosocial conditions. Thus, although rehabilitative physical therapy in a specific case can be undertaken, which is informed by medical fact and generalized experience, in terms of more general psychological development and individualized educational intervention, it becomes difficult to categorize and prescribe specifically appropriate strategies. This is especially the case if the goal is to provide early intervention in the psychological development of very young children. Such intervention is designed to promote optimum development, thus operating on a primary or secondary level of prevention, not of the handicapping condition itself, but of those socio-emotional and cognitive learning problems which, in the judgment of the interventionists, will very likely develop in association with the handicap.

Cerebral palsy, by definition, implies damage to the brain. However, damage to the motor area of the brain by no means, in itself, implies impaired conceptualization. Although approximately 50 percent of those afflicted with cerebral palsy have been estimated to have measured IQ's below seventy (within the range of mental retardation), a wide range of intellectual functioning is reported over all (Phelps, 1946).

The more specific and localized brain damage characteristic of athetosis is less likely to result in general retardation, in contrast to the spastic type where damage to the brain is generally more global (Keats, 1973). Whether an impairment in cognitive functioning is observed that is directly associated with cortical lesions is often difficult to establish, but it is improbable that damage would usually be limited specifically to motor areas.

INTELLIGENCE IN HANDICAPPED CHILDREN

The effects of physical handicaps on intellectual functioning, as measured by IQ tests, may be due to any of several factors. These include possible associated damage to the central nervous system; actual inability due to physical limitations to perform some required items in ability tests; academic retardation, associated with school time lost while homebound or hospitalized; expectancy of failure or low aspiration level due to previous experiences, and limited opportunity for the exploration of the environment which is presumed necessary for optimal cognitive growth (Telford and Sawrey, 1967). Thus, reports of studies concerning IQ levels of individuals with various forms of physical handicaps, vis-a-vis the norms of the general population, are difficult to interpret with respect to individual clinical prediction. With wide variability the rule, measured IQ levels of handicapped individuals are observed to average as much as one standard deviation below the normal mean of 100. One can make only gross probabilistic statements about predictions of cognitive functioning levels in the general and very heterogenous population of handicapped individuals, given such actuarial data.

The special problems inherent in the assessment of intellectual functioning of handicapped children have been described by Freedheim (1966) and Sattler (1973), among others. In addition to the relatively greater difficulty which a psychological examiner may have in establishing rapport, perceptual or motoric limitations related to a child's handicapping condition may render certain test items inappropriate. Such problems necessitate modification of usual testing practices and special skill on the part of the examinee.

A handicapped child is relatively more likely than is a non-handicapped child to experience developmental problems in the intellectual sphere which, in turn, is associated strongly with success in school learning tasks. Even this gross statement, however, would serve to identify the handicapped child as belonging to a group which is, in general, more vulnerable to somewhat impaired intellectual functioning and, hence, to school failure. Thus, on a similar basis to that which has identified children of urban or rural poverty environments as comprising a "target population" for early intervention for the prevention of subsequent school failure and educational equality, the physically handicapped can be likewise identified.

Are children who have a handicapping condition of a physical nature which is either congenital or incurred early in life necessarily handicapped psychologically? The question cannot be satisfactorily answered in a general way, due to the range and variation both of physical problems themselves and of home environmental influence in providing psychological support for the child.

It has often been said that every handicapped child, regardless of what his primary disability may be, is likely to be multiply handicapped. Indeed, the incidence of problems of socio-emotional adjustment problems is undoubtedly much higher among the mentally retarded population, for example, than in the non-retarded. In fact, particularly among very young children, it is often difficult to implement differential diagnosis in the case of a preschool child whose development is slow or uneven. As Jane Kessler (1966) has described, the relationship of early mental and emotional growth are actually inseparable or, more accurately, a piece or an organic unity. Although it is often observed that Piaget has not dealt with the affective side of child development, it is his position also that "thinking" and "feeling" must be seen as a unity, subservient to development (Piaget, 1967).

In the course of the previous discussion concerning cerebral palsy, it was noted that this condition does carry with it a higher probability of impaired intellectual functioning than the general population. It was also noted, however, that lower performance on measures of intellectual functioning, IQ tests, may be associated with any of a variety of factors in these children. Where there is organic brain damage, however, as is by definition the case with cerebral palsy, there is greater likelihood of impaired cognitive functioning, depending at least in part on the extent of injury. In many instances, damage to the motor area of the brain may be one manifestation of a more generalized impairment, with etiology associated with anoxia at the time of birth or other cause.

In a classic study of relationships between motor handicaps and "personality" variables, in this case integrative ideation, Wenar (1954) found severity of handicap to be significantly associated with decreased integrative ability. The task involved, called the World Test, allowed assessment of integrative abilities through their reflection in item category usage in constructing a "world" using a variety of miscellaneous items. However, despite the statistically significant differences found between non-handicapped eight to ten-year-old children, those with mild handicaps, and those with severe handicaps, Wenar noted the high incidence of overlap among the three groups. In addition, Wenar noted no evidence of a relationship between motor handicap and deviate thinking.

Investigating figure-ground disturbance in children with all forms of cerebral palsy, Dolphin and Cruickshank (1951) confirmed their hypothesis that these children, following the pattern described by Strauss and Lehtinen (1947), would have difficulty distinguishing figure from ground. This disturbance was regarded by Strauss and Lehtinen as one of the major manifestations of a syndrome of organic brain injury, subsequently termed the "Strauss Syndrome." This view drew an association between figure-background disturbance, a perceptual problem, and chronic inability to inhibit movement, vulnerability to extraneous stimulation, and other characteristics frequently observed in the neurologically handicapped child.

INTELLIGENCE AND DEVELOPMENT

It must be noted that the concept of intelligence can be viewed in various ways. Common popular and professional usage identifies intelligence as a characteristic, or a trait or trait cluster, on the basis of which individuals can be distinguished from each other or grouped together because of their commonality. In this sense, intelligence is an individual difference construct. Individuals can be indentified as functioning on a specified level with respect to intelligence, and this identification is normally accomplished through administration of a test purporting to measure the characteristic. The preceding discussion, relative to the performance of handicapped individuals on intelligence measures and their resulting IQ scores, reflects this usage.

However, intelligence as the term is used by Piaget has a different meaning. Piaget has appeared less interested in individual differences in manifestations of intelligence at some particular developmental level than the commonality of behaviors evincing intellection and the universality of the processes inferred to underlie those behaviors. Intelligence is, in this sense, a *basic process* construct. This distinction appears significant in light of tendencies to equate "cognitive" intervention programs for young children with attempts to boost IQ, tendencies to which many professionals react with pessimism or with distaste. Although it is possible to infer from Piaget's work, as J. McV. Hunt (1961) and other eminent psychologists as well as educators have done, evidence for the potential impact of enriched early experience on rate of cognitive growth and even IQ, Piaget himself has expressed little interest in such questions (Ginsburg and Opper, 1969).

In the conceptualization of Project HEED, the developmental intervention program described in this book, and more especially in its on-going, day-to-day implementation, the attempt was made to apply general positions inferred from Piaget's work. These positions included such principles as the following: the child is an active agent throughout the course of his cognitive growth; the relation between child and environment is one of mutual transaction; an important role must be accorded generic accomplishments, including object permanence, physical causality, object relations in physical space, and the operation of epistemic curiosity and the need to resolve perceptual incongruity are pervasive sources of intrinsic motivation for intellectual development.

It was assumed that these principles apply in the development of thinking in handicapped children as they do in the nonhandicapped. If the epigenesis of thought occurs naturally when the organism is intact and the environment is not deprived, where either of these conditions may not be fully met, it was assumed that external intervention is indicated as a means of promoting, for example, tactile manipulation of objects, imitation by the child of acts performed by others and especially imitation of acts performed by the child himself.

In Piaget's theoretical framework, sequential progress through six substages of sensorimotor functioning, culminating in specified generic attainments and capabilities, usher in representational functions and eventually make possible, once again to use David Elkind's phrase, "the conquest of the symbol" (Elkind, 1970). It is thus appropriate in identifying points of interest in the cognitive function of children two and three years of age, irrespective of age-equivalency scores on intelligence, perceptual, motor, or language scales, to focus on certain general areas of concern. Does the child imitate an act performed by an adult? Does his overt behavior demonstrate intent to achieve a desired end in the physical environment? Does his behavior indicate an awareness of cause-effect relationships, an ability to make predictions concerning environmental events, a disposition to formulate and to test "motor hypotheses"? Does the child play, and with what materials, and in what fashion? Does he demonstrate an awareness of self and of others as distinct from him?

It is obvious that such abilities as these are indeed tapped by infant intelligence scales, such as the Cattell Infant Scales (1940) employed in Project HEED for initial and periodic assessment. One child may be manifesting relatively "more" intelligence than another, and a child may show progress or increased attainment relative to test norms as an interactive function of maturation and learning. What must be noted, however, is that the score alone may be of less interest and have fewer implications for how to teach the child than careful observations of what that child does in relation to his physicosocial environment. Such observations may be of great value whether conducted in specific task situations, such as a test administration or teacher-presented task, or in the natural flow of events in a classroom or other setting. In general, the former situation requires that observation be conducted without external intervention, or "teaching," whereas the latter may involve an adult in the facilitation of a discovery or the modification of an act. It may be noted that Piaget's *clinical method*, essentially a child-centered interview or questioning procedure, permits the adult some latitude for "nondirective" involvement with the child in a situation, and for relatively open-ended assessment, following the lead suggested by each response made by the child.

In the subsequent discussion of the goals formulated and the strategies implemented in Project HEED, it will be seen that observation of each child in the course of his participation in the program played a major role. As guides for observation, staff relied on several sources. These included, in addition to the professional experience of each individual as a clinician and the tutelage of his own discipline, theoretical propositions concerning early psychological development such as those described in the foregoing discussion.

Based on Piaget's work, Drs. Ina C. Uzgiris and J. McV. Hunt (1964) have developed a series of ordinal scales for assessing the developmental progress of infants in six areas of sensorimotor functioning:

(1) Visual pursuit and permanence of objects
(2) Means for achieving desired environmental events
(3) Gestural and vocal imitation
(4) Operational causality
(5) Object relations in space
(6) Schemas for relating to objects

Previous discussion in this chapter, it is hoped, has served to illustrate the relevance of each of these areas to the experience of young children whose physical development is exceptional, i.e. whose interaction with the physical environment is in any way impeded by a limiting or handicapping condition during the first two years of life. The project was not undertaken to test hypotheses relative to this position, however; rather, it was believed that the work of Piaget could serve to provide a framework both for observing and for facilitating the cognitive growth processes of participating children.

Through the course of its rather brief history as a scientific discipline, the psychology of human development has generated a great many research findings of relevance to intervention projects such as that to be described in the following chapters. As William Rohwer (1971) has written, there continue to be four major issues which perennially produce controversy and, consequently, stimulate inquiry: heredity vs. environment; maturation vs. learning; stages vs. continuous development, and critical periods. All of these issues are of vital importance in Project HEED; indeed, they are to any attempt at early intervention as a means to influence in some way the course of subsequent development for young children.

Surprisingly, in the field of special education, studies concerning "early influences" on the psychological development of children with motor handicaps seem to have produced few conclusive findings and firm guides for action. Concepts from the psychology of "normal" child development, such as competence, autonomy, and self-concept, and the general theoretical perspectives of Piaget and of Erikson concerning early development of intelligence and self were believed to bear a special significance and to offer particular usefulness when applied to young children with marked physical handicaps.

CHAPTER 3

PROJECT HEED:
PURPOSES AND RATIONALE

CONTEXT OF THE PROJECT:
CONTEMPORARY EARLY CHILDHOOD EDUCATION

RECENT YEARS HAVE WITNESSED considerable ferment in education in general, with new thrusts in the directions of improving educational opportunity for the poor, humanizing education for all learners, using technology effectively, and substituting relevance for mindlessness (Silberman, 1970). No areas of education, however, have received more attention during this current period in the form of innovative approaches, manpower training and effective utilization, rigorous experimentation and evaluation, and heightened public awareness than those of special education and early childhood education. Yet most individuals acquainted with either of these fields would agree that with respect to both, only bare beginnings have been realized.

The domain of special education is continuously being redefined and expanded. New concepts such as *educationally handicapped* and *non-categorical programs* have emerged as educators have attempted to adapt medical, sociological, psychological, and legal phenomena to educationally relevant language.

In terms of the concerns of special education, the education of young children has several salient features: (1) especially adapted instruction for young children who are exceptional, or handicaped; (2) identification and screening of children who will potentially become educationally handicapped upon entering school, and (3) primary prevention of educational handicaps, i.e. problems in school learning and/or social behavior in the school setting.

Vehicles for the provision of special education, initially restricted essentially to special schools, special class placement within regular school, and tutoring for homebound or hospitalized children, have similarly increased in number and ingenuity. Crisis teachers, helping teachers, teacher-counselors, "teaching moms," resource rooms, and still other adaptations have been created to assist the school-age child. For the handicapped child of kindergarten age or younger, program options including enriched kindergarten programs, special or therapeutic nursery schools and kindergartens, and parent education and casework counseling have been provided.

Practically all of these special education program designs for young handicapped children are restricted to children three years of age or older. It must also be noted that, on a nationwide basis, very few of the three to five-year-old children with physical, intellectual, or emotional problems who would be eligible for such programs are enrolled. The vast majority of handicapped children who are identified as special education candidates are not so identified until their first school failures and other school problems begin to occur. Even beyond that point, however, it is commonly estimated that more than one-half of the American school children with serious handicaps do not receive special educational assistance, including supportive services for maintenance, in the mainstream of the regular classroom environment.

The other side of this coin of identification, labeling and stigmatization is particularly likely to affect the child whose handicapping condition is highly visible. The problem of school exclusion has been recognized in recent years as a central concern shared by general and special educators, and is increasingly coming into national prominence as an issue of constitutionality and civil rights. For example, whether a school district can meet its legal requirements of providing for the education of a child confined to a wheelchair by making possible enrollment in a special school will undoubtedly be increasingly subject to challenge. If the child's best interests would be served by allowing him to pursue his schooling in integrated fashion with non-handicapped peers, it may be that a school's two or three story construction, for example, will not be regarded as a legitimate excuse for refusing regular school placement.

Recent intense interest is at least in part related to the general question retarding education and schooling raised during the 1960's: Can education compensate for the problems of society? Social ills such as racism and sexism, discrimination and segregation, crime, violence and militarism, marital and family instability, and poverty and unemployment have been identified as targets for educational reformers. Social ills in terms of individual adjustment and personal-social competence include alcoholism and drug abuse, delinquency and alienation, learning disturbance, emotional disorders, and, most recently, unethical conduct.

Whether the concern is *To Change a Child* (Powledge, 1967), or to change the society via the socializing institutions, young children have been assumed to be more amenable to external influence. Based in part on the truism, "As the twig is bent, so grows the tree," and on the traditional Freudian belief that personality is quite well established by age five or six, recent efforts in early childhood education have proliferated.

Regarding the issue of intellectual functioning and learning capability, two highly influential books appeared in the early 1960's which gave impetus to the compensatory educational programs for young children which were soon to burgeon. In *Intelligence and Experience* (1961) J. McV. Hunt dealt extensively with the traditional nativism vs. empiricism battle as it relates to human intellectual development. Reviewing the evidence and drawing support from the work of Piaget and the neuropsychological theory of Donald Hebb (1949), Hunt made a strong case for the malleability of human intelligence. In *Stability and Change in Human Characteristics*, Benjamin S. Bloom (1964) concluded from his exhaustive review of the research literature that levels of intellectual functioning at adulthood can be fairly effectively predicted by the time children have reached school, with a level of accuracy considerably surpassing chance. The younger the child, however, the more tenuous the prediction, leading to the inference that intellectual functioning may be far more amenable to influence during the early childhood years. Bloom further proposed the hypothesis that human abilities may be most susceptible to environmental, experiential influence during their periods of most rapid growth.

Whether the early childhood years would comprise *critical periods* for the development of general functions or specific behaviors has not actually been resolved. However, the sense of urgency associated with early childhood intervention efforts in the 1960's was very pronounced, as exemplified by books such as *Revolution in Learning* by Maya Pines (1966).

Thus, armed with a theoretical base and scientific support, Project Head Start began with much hope and promise as a major arm of the national War on Poverty. Despite enthusiastic support in many quarters and numerous reports of success, the ubiquitous IQ soon began to appear rather less tractable than had initially appeared to be the case. With some very notable exceptions (Weikart, *et al.*, 1970), the interventionists appeared to be plagued again by the problem of developmental regression.

Attempts to deal with this problem have proceeded in several directions, some of them overlapping:

1. Questioning what schools may do to children—whether the subsequent deleterious effects of schooling may be so severe for some children as to preclude the possibility of inoculating them against failure.
2. Questioning the viability of IQ as a salient criterion variable.
3. Initiating Project Follow Through to extend the impact of Head Start into the first regular school years.
4. Experimenting with alternative program designs, both in Head Start and Follow Through.
5. Moving toward earlier intervention, even infant programs.
6. Moving toward more comprehensive intervention, especially through involvement of parents (usually mothers) in the programs.

The last two points listed above have been manifest in such programs as Parent and Child Centers and Project Home Start. In general, there are two models: center based programs and home based programs. In both cases, however, the goal is to help the parent to become a more effective teacher of her infant or young child by being more aware of the child as a rapidly learning individual and by interacting with him in positive, stimulating, and growth-inducing ways.

Two of these current trends have been incorporated in the conceptualization and implementation of Project HEED:

1. The trend toward earlier and more comprehensive intervention.
2. The trend toward increased involvement of mothers as a central focus for intervention.

As an attempt at early intervention on behalf of young children with marked physical handicaps, Project HEED must be seen within the context of current patterns in American education. Early education, i.e. structured, formalized learning experiences for pre-school children, has during recent years, been influenced most notably by new efforts to promote the optimal development of the children of the poor.

However, the concepts of *early intervention* and *primary* and *secondary prevention* have been and continue to be related to the teaching of children at any socio-economic level. In the mental health fields, these concepts are associated with the prevention of emotional or behavioral disturbance, mental illness, psychopathy and a sense of alienation. Viewed more positively, they relate to the promotion of effective functioning, social responsibility, a sense of personal well-being, and the realization of human potential.

Project HEED, though focusing on the special needs of children who have pronounced medical problems, most of which are at the present time not reversible or remediable *per se*, was conceived within the framework of early education as an ameliorative and positive influence in the lives of young children.

RATIONALE: THE CONCEPTS OF EARLY INTERVENTION AND
PRIMARY AND SECONDARY PREVENTION

The position is taken here that all education is undertaken in order to effect some change in the course of children's development, that is, to influence development so that its rate, sequence, or quality is different as a consequence of the experience. Every educational program thus represents an intent to intervene in the lives of children so as to promote the achievement of some desirable goal.

The rationale for early intervention, as has been pointed out, is rooted in assumptions, theories, and inferences drawn from empirical research findings and is intimately tied to the environmentalist rather than the maturationist position. Based in part on Bloom's conclusion (1964) that human abilities may be most vulnerable to external influence during their periods of most rapid growth, most early intervention programs stress the important strides made during the early years in areas such as language acquisition. From traditional Freudian personality theory comes the view, perhaps an overly deterministic one, that patterns of personality and character development are usually well established during the years before formal schooling begins. A child's self-concept, too, of his own value to others, his competence, his similarity to admired and loved parents, is assumed to be rooted in very early experiences.

The concept of primary prevention is borrowed from the field of mental health (see, for example, Caplan, 1961). Early educational experiences can serve as a preventive force, it is assumed, in ways such as:

1. Helping a child to acquire a diverse range of avenues for impulse gratification.
2. Enabling the child to acquire the expectancy of success in school and social situations, in order to set into a motion a positive, rather than negative, self-fulfilling prophecy.
3. Enabling the child to develop a range of means for coping with stressful situations in his physical and social world.
4. Helping the child to acquire basic skills and understandings upon which later learning can be built, thus making successful learning more likely in the future.
5. Promoting a positive "set" toward school, toward learning, teachers, peers, and himself.
6. Helping the child to acquire patterns of behavior which will be acceptable to peers and adults in school and elsewhere.

7. Helping the child to understand his own feelings and those of others and to acquire both personal responsibility for his own behavior and empathy and understanding concerning the behavior of others.

Project HEED can be seen, then, as a program designed to provide primary and secondary prevention through early intervention for handicapped children. It is not supposed that the handicapping condition can be eliminated through early developmental education. The rehabilitative focus, emphasis, and tradition of the agency, as well as the limitations in current medical knowledge and, perhaps, the inevitable irreversibility of certain physical problems, all dictate the following as a major objective for this program: *to assist the child in attaining the most effective functioning possible within the limits imposed by his handicap*.

Prevention is an appropriate concept in this instance when applied to (1) functional developmental disabilities associated with an organic and essentially irreversible handicap; (2) eventual disabilities in personal and social adjustment, acceptance, and adaptation to which handicapped children are believed to be especially vulnerable, and (3) disabilities or problems in the acquisition of basic academic skills when these children undertake formal schooling.

With respect to the last area, it is accepted that rehabilitation, rather than prevention, will in many instances be the more realistic goal. For example, many children with cerebral palsy, despite language and cognitive competence, may lack the fine motor control to write adequately. For such a child, eventual training in the use of a typewriter often proves an invaluable asset, enabling him to function quite competently within the regular educational milieu.

BACKGROUND: THE CHILDREN AND THE AGENCY

Two-year-old children were ineligible to participate in the nursery school program conducted by The Society for Crippled Children of Cuyahoga County. Moreover, this program, as it was constituted, was inappropriate to the needs of these very young children, many of whom were not ambulatory, had not yet acquired speech, and were not yet capable of even rudimentary self-care. It was felt, however, that such children were not too young to benefit from an educational program if it were especially tailored to their needs.

The nursery school for handicapped children admitted many children at age three. However, by age two the effects of physical handicaps are already causing retardation of social and emotional development in many children. Unless the two-year-old can begin to gain mastery over his body and its functions, his entire personality may, according to generally accepted theory, be affected.

The child with a severe physical handicap is often denied the experience of relating to peers. Because his development proceeds neither at the same rate nor in the same manner as that of the nonhandicapped child, he is often infantilized by his parents. His days are spent in an adult world of parents, doctors, nurses, and therapists. He therefore lacks the opportunity for interactions with other children and, consequently, for the learning which is inherent in such exposure. The opportunity for a small-group learning experience was suggested as a means for providing these early social interactions.

Project HEED was preceeded by a pilot program called the Developmental Group. As a forerunner of the present project it provided a learning experience for the staff; therefore, a brief description of its inception, physical layout, staff and philosophy is helpful in understanding the objectives and methodology of the present program.

THE PILOT PROJECT

Two-year-old Joan cried unceasingly every Monday morning. That was the day every week that her mother brought her to the agency for the physical therapy treatment prescribed by her physician. Even after a year of regular visits her entrance through the front door was heralded by screams of protest.

Shortly after her third birthday Joan entered the Heman

Nursery School. The teachers were fully prepared to help her cope with a difficult adjustment period. They anticipated that her mother's presence would be required for many days, perhaps weeks, before she would be reassured and able to accept the two teachers assigned to her class, the new classroom surroundings and her eleven classmates. Within the first week Joan no longer needed her mother to accompany her to school. She had quickly transferred trust to her teachers, cautiously investigated the new setting and even cooperated in her physical therapy treatment without a whimper.

Joan was one of many children who followed much the same pattern, and the staff examined the factors involved for the child as an outpatient and then as a member of the nursery school. The most obvious difference was age: three years of age as compared to two. However, even as the child approached her third birthday she tended to remain tense and anxious during her therapy visits. It seemed apparent that children might benefit from a setting less threatening than the physical therapy room, a room equipped with toys and materials appealing to and appropriate for the very young child, a setting, in fact, similar to a nursery school classroom. To provide for the children's need for comfort and security and to ensure a meaningful follow-through home program, mothers were to be included in each session. This kind of setting would afford an ideal opportunity to institute a comprehensive early education program, one that would encourage the accomplishment of developmental tasks and stimulate the acquisition of cognitive and linguistic skills which are often hampered as a consequence of physical handicaps.

The intention of the pilot project was not necessarily to accelerate the child's learning rate but to enable him to gain sufficient mastery of his body so that he could explore his environment and begin to acquire greater awareness of self and independence. It was anticipated that along with these gains would come decreased frustration and increased ability and motivation in cognitive areas. As the physical environment was broadened and enriched, the child could be expected to develop a greater degree of self-awareness and an increased awareness of his ability to make an impact on his environment and thereby to develop a sense of competence.

The supervisors of three departments, Nursery School, Physical Therapy, and Social Service, formulated plans for the Developmental Group, as it was named. The Nursery School Supervisor coordinated the program and planned age appropriate activities for the children. The group was scheduled to meet one morning a week for two hours, with a teacher and physical therapist assigned to the children and a caseworker available to the parents for group sessions and individual counseling.

A corner of the staff conference room was the only space available. It contained a sofa, several comfortable chairs, and an expanse of carpeted floor. Three small square tables and eight chairs borrowed from the nursery school provided the furniture required for the children. Dolls, small wheeled vehicles, musical instruments, puzzles, formboards, paints and crayons were donated by the employees of a local industrial firm.

The parents of eight two-year-old children who were being treated in the physical therapy department were contacted by the social service supervisor who explained the new program, and all were eager to participate.

Because fear, anger and unwillingness to separate from the mother had served as a deterrent to successful therapy sessions, it was necessary to minimize and, if possible, to eliminate the circumstances producing the stress. A tense, crying child who refuses to be comforted often elicits embarrassment in the mother who, in turn, transmits further tension and uneasiness to the child. To facilitate the child's coping with unfamiliar surroundings and new adults, the first few sessions in the new program were completely unstructured. Mothers spent this time playing with their children, offering them a new toy, and showing them what to do with it. The teacher and physical therapist were available to mothers and children to help when needed, but primarily to permit the children an opportunity to become accustomed to them. This unstructured, relaxed beginning allowed the mothers time to become acquainted with the other mothers and their children as well as with the staff. It was a time for further explanation of the new program and its philosophy and goals.

After the first few sessions most of the children were able to separate from their mothers to teacher or therapist for brief periods. Mothers gathered in the kitchen across the hall for coffee, group sessions, or just to chat, but were always available to return to their children when needed. As the children began to adjust to separation from their mothers, the teacher introduced new toys and encouraged exploration and investigation as the physical therapist resumed therapy treatments within the room. Within a month the mothers requested that the group meet twice a week because of their children's response to the program and their own desire for additional contact with staff and each other.

As changes in a child's behavior occurred and were interpreted to the mother who, as an active participant, had shared the experience with the child and staff, she began increasingly to view her handicapped child as capable of learning and herself as capable of teaching him. Role models were provided by teachers and therapists to enable parents to learn ways of interacting with their children which would enhance the child's development. It is often noted by professionals working with handicapped children that their mothers suffer from a lack of feedback. Stages of development extend over longer periods of time and changes occur so gradually that mothers often feel their efforts are unrewarded. A child who accepts spoon feeding early, albeit sloppily, rewards his mother beyond the time and effort she expends in the process. A repeated gagging reflex and frustrated cries, on the other hand, may elicit in the mother feelings of inadequacy, and after numerous unsuccessful experiences with a resistant child, her response may be to return to bottle feeding the child. One of the principal functions of both teacher and therapist was to encourage the mothers by example to continue to work toward realistic goals and to recognize limited but gradual progress along the way. A mother who feels capable of fostering her child's development gains a sense of her own parenting competence and a more satisfying feedback.

Often parents of exceptional children feel a sense of isolation. This program afforded the opportunity for identification
and mutual support with other parents of handicapped children. As mothers shared their feelings of guilt, often themselves assuming blame for the child's deficits, the others in the
group pointed out how unrealistic these feelings were. In informal unplanned encounters they passed along management
techniques and information concerning uses of equipment.

These mothers reported gaining a sense of solidarity as a
result of meeting other parents of handicapped children and
by sharing mutual concerns and anxieties. Because their
children's developmental patterns had differed from those of
friends' and neighbors' children, many of the parents had
experienced a sense of alienation. They were often at a loss to
understand or explain the child's needs and consequently had
felt inadequate to provide proper parenting. In the group
sessions they spoke of their frustrations and expressed
gratitude at having met each other.

One morning a mother arrived late looking unwell and com-
plaining of a headache. However, she had refused to miss the
session and reported that her husband had complimented her
on being a good mother. She then confided to the group, "I'm
not doing this just for Billie, I'm doing it for me too."

As the year progressed, parents continued to come despite
weather and travel conditions, and gains in social and motor
skills among the children became increasingly apparent.

PROGRAM OBJECTIVES AND PROGRAM DESIGN

Through a foundation grant the agency was able to make
plans to formalize and enlarge the program for the following
year.

Although the staff observed and reported gains in socialization, motor, and language skills, no formal documentation had
been undertaken other than descriptive anecdotal reports. An
evaluation design was incorporated in Project HEED in order
to determine to what extent and in what areas program objectives were met.

General objectives for the program, children, and the parents remained basically the same as they had been in the pilot program.

To enable the children to:

1. Accomplish the developmental tasks of body mastery so as to gain a sense of competence, gain ability and inclination to explore the environment, and gain a degree of independence, tasks common to handicapped and nonhandicapped children.
2. Achieve greater self-awareness and more positive self-evaluation.
3. Achieve a higher degree of readiness for the demands of the regular nursery school and special therapies program.
4. Attain a higher degree of security regarding separation from the mother.
5. Gain experience in a peer-group setting.
6. Gain experience in interacting with adults in teaching roles.
7. Attain cognitive and linguistic learning (such as symbolic functioning and representational thought) which may be hampered as a consequence of a physical handicap.

To enable the parents to:

1. View their children as learners and themselves as teachers, as well as mothers.
2. Imitate and learn from role models provided by teachers and therapists ways of interacting with their children which may enhance development.
3. Express and share their feelings as parents of handicapped children and thereby gain a sense of solidarity and mutual support.
4. Gain a greater sense of their ability to foster their children's learning and development in spite of their handicaps.

THE INTERDISCIPLINARY TEAM

Staff had been made available to the Developmental Group in the pilot project either by being excused from their regular duties in the agency or by assuming additional responsibilities in order to participate in the program. A teacher from the nursery school had been responsible for one weekly session and university graduate students in Early Childhood Education had completed a practicum assignment through working with the project staff one day each week. The caseworker had increased her normal caseload to provide counseling to parents in the Developmental Group. The foundation grant now made it possible to engage staff whose responsibilities five mornings each week are specifically to the parents and children enrolled in Project HEED.

In the design for Project HEED, a physical therapist, a teacher and a teacher's assistant were to be the constants in the classroom. The physical therapist is responsible for planning and implementing each child's therapy program according to his individual needs. The teacher's function is to guide each child in the acquisition of cognitive and linguistic skills by encouraging age-appropriate activities within the limits imposed by the medical problem. Together teacher and physical therapist carry out therapy and educational goals in a group setting utilizing skill building and creative materials and gross motor equipment. The teacher, with the aid of her assistant, is responsible for the selection and maintenance of all materials and equipment. She coordinates and integrates into the daily activities suggestions of all therapists and consultants. In addition, the teacher maintains a daily record of each child's progress.

In the Developmental Group, physical therapy had taken place within the setting but had been accomplished basically on a one-to-one basis between therapist and child. In Project HEED, however, greater emphasis was to be placed on integrating therapy with education-play activities.

The occupational therapist, speech pathologist and psychologist recommend immediate and long-range goals for each child and offer suggestions for specific activities to be incorporated. They also administer periodic evaluations and assessments which are described in Chapter 4.

The caseworker holds one weekly parent session for each

group and is available for individual counseling as it is requested or required. She shares with the staff working directly with the children any pertinent information which may provide insight into the child's behavior or prove helpful in planning. Although initial intake is the responsibility of the agency casework supervisor, the HEED caseworker is the primary liaison person between the mother and child and the HEED staff.

ISSUES AND PROBLEMS IN PROGRAM EVALUATION

Project HEED was conceived, funded, and implemented primarily to serve two general aims: (1) to provide direct service to very young physically handicapped children and to their families (becoming thus an extension of the previously existing agency program), and (2) to demonstrate the feasibility and viability of an innovative approach having the following components:

1. early ameliorative intervention for young handicapped children (modal age, two years)
2. multidisciplinary team approach
3. provision of individualized education and special therapies within the group setting
4. group, as opposed to one-to-one, approach
5. center-based, as opposed to home-based, program
6. direct involvement of parents in their children's program
7. individualized casework counseling with parents
8. group-work with parents

Project objectives explicitly stated relate to three major areas: (1) Program objectives, which pertain mainly to the demonstration nature of the project and which, to some extent, presuppose success with respect to attainment of the other objectives; (2) objectives for the children, and (3) objectives for the parents. Each of the objectives within these sets can, in turn, be classified as either a process objective or an outcome objective. Process objectives are statements of intended program components (e.g. children will gain experience in a peer group setting, or a team approach will be used), and must be dealt with conscientiously in evaluating the program. In some instances, these can provide extremely objective and useful information. Occasionlly, something that was promised in a proposal does not take place. Every human services agency and program can be held, or holds itself, accountable for the attainment of process objectives. Reporting of the number of treatment hours provided, the number of patients, clients, or students served, the components of a curriculum or program reflects such accountability.

Process objectives, however, do not in themselves specify what will happen as a result of the services described. They do not deal with issues such as whether a client, patient, or student was benefited from the service, whether he could have realized the same benefits had he not received the services, or whether he is different in any way than if he had not participated.

Many service programs, operating on the basis of assumptions which may or may not be supported by theoretical grounding and/or empirical knowledge, rely primarily on process objectives. Or, if outcome objectives are stated, they may be either untested or untestable. Educational curricula and methods provide numerous examples. Often, outcome behaviors may indeed be specified and measured, but these may fail to represent accurate or complete criterion measures in light of the stated aims and purposes of the program. In fields such as psychotherapy, objectives must often be stated in such individualistic and conditional terms that both prediction of "success" and evaluation of outcome are extremely difficult and tenuous. (This is not the case for behavior therapists who state outcome objectives in terms of specific client behaviors.)

In connection with the stated outcome objectives for Project HEED, the staff was aware of some potential dangers and limitations inherent in the nature of the program:

1. Criterion performance levels within any area will vary as a function of individual child characteristics (e.g., level of entering behavior).
2. Target areas for intervention will vary as a function of individual child needs and staff resources.

(These two limitations simply imply that individualized outcome objectives for each child must be specified.)

3. It is possible that measured gains in nearly any outcome performance measure may be unstable over time, due to such phenomena as normal statistical regression and spurious and shortlived treatment effects.

4. It is also possible that treatment effects may not be immediately apparent and/or may take some form other than that predicted.

5. Scales administered as measures of outcome objectives can only approximate and provide inferences concerning real world behavior.

6. It is difficult to specify the ways in which program components (treatment variables) will interact with child characteristics to produce certain outcomes—or indeed, to specify what will constitute "treatment" for each individual child.

As an early intervention program for young physically handicapped and multiply handicapped children, Project HEED could draw from the experiences of a variety of programs and professional disciplines. Just as early education and development efforts undertaken with children from disadvantaged backgrounds have during recent years been increasingly guided by psychological theory concerning cognitive and socio-emotional growth, so the staff of this project recognized the universality of principles and processes of development operative in these young handicapped children. The methods of intervention used in work both with children and with parents were grounded in theory, as well as in the pragmatic demands of reality situations and issues. Most of the remaining chapters are devoted to the discussion of these methods and their rationale.

CHAPTER 4

THE FORMATIVE EVALUATION PROCESS

RELATIVE TO THE EVALUATION of the impact of a program on the children involved, it is one thing to attempt to relate observed gains in the children to effects of the program, rather than simply maturation, but quite another matter to detect interactive relationships between specific program aspects and specific areas of behavior demonstrated by individual children.

What was of central interest, given a rather heterogenous group of physically handicapped two-year-old children, was not the general issue of the efficacy of intervention vs. no intervention. The position was taken that the question of whether gains would or would not have occurred had the child not been enrolled in the program would have to be dealt with idiographically in the case of each child. Beyond that, it was believed that information of a much more specific nature than whether the overall effect of the program had been beneficial would be obtainable. The staff hoped to document observable behavior changes as they occurred and to attempt to relate such changes to identifiable program components.

It was also assumed that such documentation would serve the primary function of guiding work with the child as an individual. This position acknowledges two fundamental principles of working with children in a treatment situation: (1) what may at times become a trial-and-error approach, informed by case-specific empirical observation, as characterized by a continuing process of hypothesis formulation and testing, is an appropriate and usually necessary style, and (2) objectives, once established, need continuously to be re-examined and replaced, when appropriate, by new objectives. Each of these principles relates to the more general rule that a child is a constantly changing organism. What is true today, what predictions would seem tenable today, may be greatly altered with the passage of time, the course of biological maturation, and with exposure to new environmental contingencies.

Beyond the medical realities of a handicapping condition, the psychological realities vary widely from individual to individual. The child's response to limited mobility will be determined by many of the wide variety of individual characteristics which affect the behavior of all children. These variables, including such attributes as exploratory curiosity, perseverance, self-valuation, responsiveness to the social environment, and the like were assumed to be at least in part amenable to experiential influence.

The apparently very important influence of home environment on the subsequent adjustment of the child with a physical handicap was noted earlier. A role of central importance was assigned to the parent component of Project HEED, which is discussed in detail in subsequent chapters, including a description of evaluation strategies employed.

DIAGNOSIS AND TEAM PLANNING

Although objectives had been formulated which would presumably apply to all children involved in the project, it yet remained to cast those objectives in operational form for each individual child. In effect, a treatment plan had to be devised by the interdisciplinary team for each child, one based on specific diagnostic information obtained for individuals within the framework of the project objectives.

The need at this point was for a coordinated initial diagnostic study of each child by the team, a study that would point toward attainable short-term and long-term goals. It was believed essential that this diagnostic study be orchestrated, rather than fragmented, with a coordinated focus of clinical disciplines on the whole child. The absolute necessity of effective communication among team members was insisted upon from the beginning.

An unfortunate tendency in many clinical settings serving children with special problems, whether of a physical or psychiatric nature, is for a clinical discipline to establish its claim to a part of the child and to jealously guard its function. Children, however, engage in fine motor control activity whether with an occupational therapist or a teacher, practice body positioning with or without a physical therapist and may acquire shape concepts in the company of anyone, not only the teacher. Motor activity, peer interaction, and observing interesting events outdoors through the window may be accompanied by speech, whether observed, recorded, and facilitated by the language therapist or by anyone else. Thus, although each team member brought to the project specific competencies and areas of specific interest, these were contributed to a unified team effort.

In addition, Project HEED was conceived not only as a means of providing direct intervention for children through the services of a team of specialists, but also indirect intervention through enhancing the abilities of parents of these children to foster their development. Even beyond this, however, the parent was regarded as a direct recipient of service. No effort on behalf of the child could be considered apart form the parent or parents involved. It was assumed that the well-being of parents and child were inseparable, and that meaningful impact of the program on the child would be contingent upon the parent.

The means of determining objectives realizable through the program for participating parents as agency clients was social casework study. Such study was developmental, beginning with the gathering of referral materials and comprehensive intake interviews, and continuing through the modes of individual case counseling and group work. An indispensable factor in Project HEED was the contribution of all team members to the caseworker's understanding of the parents in relation to their child and as individuals in their own right. Conversely, every team member's interaction with a parent was informed by the caseworker's understanding of the total picture presented by the needs of that parent and those of the total family group. Again, although project objectives suggested the areas within which help for parents would be offered, the specificity of each parent's and each family's situation determined individual objectives and strategies.

It was determined to conduct an initial coordinated diagnostic assessment of each child's functioning which could be repeated at six month intervals. This procedure was intended to serve two major functions: to provide an objective standard for evaluating program impact on each individual child and on the group as a whole, and to provide guidance for individualized intervention in specific areas by noting specific strengths and weaknesses. Each discipline then presented its findings in a diagnostic staff conference held for each child, at which time congruent and dissonant observations were thoroughly discussed and resolved, the goal being the establishment of a unified treatment plan for each child.

Even before this, and continuously throughout the diagnostic staffings, the effort to set objectives for individuals was related to overall program objectives. This served to keep the team constantly aware of the principle that goals established for individual children cut across the boundaries of professional disciplines, and that closely coordinated effort was needed to achieve these goals. They were first stated as areas toward which work with children would be directed; appropriate evaluation techniques were matched with them.

OBJECTIVES FOR THE CHILDREN

Objective	*Method of Assessment*
1. Accomplish age-appropriate developmental tasks	
a. Body mastery	Motor Development Test Occupational Therapy Evaluation
b. Sense of competence	Cattell Infant Scales Preschool Attainment Record
c. Exploration of environment	Vineland Scales Teacher's Periodic Checklist

Objective:	Method of Assessment:
d. Independence (individuation, autonomy)	Teacher's Daily Record
2. Achieve self-awareness and positive self-evaluation	Teacher's Periodic Checklist Teacher's Daily Record
3. Achieve readiness for nursery school and therapy programs of agency	Teacher's Periodic Checklist Summative assessments, all therapists
4. Attain security regarding separation	Teacher's Periodic Checklist Teacher's Daily Record
5. Gain experience in peer setting	Teacher's Periodic Checklist Teacher's Daily Record
6. Gain experience with adults in teaching role	Teacher's Periodic Checklist Teacher's Daily Record Summative assessments, all therapists
7. Attain cognitive and linguistic learning	
a. Symbolic play	Teacher's Periodic Checklist
b. Language functions: receptive	Houston Test REEL Teacher's Periodic Checklist
c. Language functions: expressive	Houston Test REEL Teacher's Periodic Checklist
d. Imitation	Teacher's Periodic Checklist Teacher's Daily Record
e. Object permanence	Cattell Infant Scales
f. Causality	Cattell Infant Scales Teacher's Periodic Checklist
g. Object schemas	Cattell Infant Scales Teacher's Periodic Checklist
h. Basic form, size, color and rational concepts	Cattell Infant Scales Vineland Scales Preschool Attainment Record Teacher's Periodic Checklist

Diagnostic procedures, intended to interface at the various objectives, were developed and implemented in the educational, language, psychological, physical therapy and occupational therapy areas.

EDUCATIONAL ASSESSMENT

The *Teacher's Periodic Checklist* is an inventory form created specifically for use with the HEED Project. It was completed by the teacher for each child immediately following the child's admission and thereafter at six month intervals. Assigned rating, with descriptive summaries, are shared with the total diagnostic and goal-setting procedure.

Areas covered by the checklist correspond to program goals formulated to direct work with the children. There are four major areas of concern:

   I. Self-awareness and Body Mastery
      A. Self-awareness
      B. Recognition of body parts
      C. Body mastery
  II. Exploration of Environment
 III. Social Adaptation
 IV. Cognitive Skills

The use of a four-point scale (0-3) permitted quantification of ratings in the form of averages in each of the areas. Of far more interest to the team, however, were the specific items themselves, for these identified observable behaviors which were amenable to observation and to the planning of intervention strategies for specific children. Each item is rated in terms of whether the behavior is consistently, often, rarely, or never present.

Self-awareness items were those which staff felt indicated the degree to which a child had a firm sense of his own identity, and included the following: (the child) recognizes own name, vocally identifies self; recognizes full-view mirror reflection of self; recognizes own photograph when it is presented together with photograph of another child; recognizes own photograph when it is presented together with several photographs of other children; asserts ownership of toys or other items; can correctly express whether he is a boy or girl.

It is apparent that some form of expressive communication is required for the performance of each of these behaviors. In view of the fact that many of the children had not progressed beyond use of one-word utterances, a number used generally unintelligible vocalizations, and a few were virtually nonvocal, the assessment procedure had to permit the child access to some alternative mode of communication. Since for the purpose of this assessment awareness of self rather than language development was of interest, every effort was made to assess the child's functioning independently of the progress of his language development or, more accurately, of his speech production level. Snatching a desired toy from the reach of an encroaching peer, for example, might suggest the presence of a sense of possession and assertion of ownership. A motor response might signal recognition of the child's name, mirror reflection, or photograph.

In *Body Part Recognition* items, the ability to point to or otherwise indicate motorically the named part is assessed. Items included the following: head, eyes, nose, mouth, ears, hands, arms, legs, feet, hair, teeth, finger-nails, tummy, shoulders.

The following *Body Mastery* items were of interest:
1. Communicates need to toilet.
2. Can feed self a cookie.
3. Can drink milk from a cup.
4. Can use tissue, handerchief, napkin.
5. Initiates gross motor activity in play.
6. Initiates fine motor activity in play.
7. Participates or assists in removing outer clothing.
8. Participates or assists in donning outer clothing.

The *Exploration of Environment* category comprises both cognitive and motivational items; the child's interest in his physical environment and his ability to interact with it and thus grow toward concept attainment were combined beneath the rubric of environmental exploration.

Item 1: Will seek desired object temporarily hidden from view. The presence of this behavior suggests the presence of the concept of the permanent object, i.e. that a child is aware of the continued independent existence of an object even though it is screened from his vision. In this important developmental achievement, knowledge and motivation go hand in hand. In working with handicapped children it is often necessary to determine whether inability to respond to this task is due primarily to motor response difficulties, lack of interest in the item, or lack of the concept itself.

Item 2: Will solicit adult assistance. Young children learn to use adults as resources in exploration, play, and important daily activities such as eating and dressing. If a child appears unable to make voluntarily affective use of adults in helping him to deal with his environment, it may reflect unsatisfactory early experiences, shyness or fear with strangers, or other cognitive-affective problems. On the other hand, the child who is so dependent on adult assistance that he is unable to function even in limited ways without it is not acquiring functional adaptive capabilities. This item reflects the reality needs of two-year-old children, especially those whose motor functioning is impaired, to be assisted by an adult in attaining some desired goal. Thus, it reflects both goal-directedness and awareness that adults can be enlisted by the child in pursuit of his goals.

Item 3: Enjoys manipulating play materials. What is of interest is evidence of enjoyment of manipulative play as a form of exploration. This sort of tactile exploratory behavior with objects is essential to what Piaget calls physical knowledge.

Item 4: Becomes absorbed in play. This item relates to the degree of involvement the child manifests in play. Although the proverbial short attention span is associated with the behavior of toddlers, children of this age are commonly observed to be deeply engrossed in play activities. Play thus takes on an intensive character, a quality to which this item has reference.

Item 5: Plays with many diverse toys and materials. The variety and extensiveness of the child's toy play repertoire, manifesting skills of both a motoric and cognitive nature, as well as range of interests and exploratory motivations, seems a useful index for examining the child's relation to his environment.

Item 6: Uses familiar objects for new purposes. Such behavior evidences a problem-solving disposition, an invention of new means for achieving desired purposes, or a willingness to experiment. Two and three-year-old children often engage in creative imaginative play with the aid of what may appear to adults unlikely materials or props.

Item 7: Within limits imposed by handicap, moves about in physical space. That a child moves about the physical environment as much as he is actually able suggests the presence of motivation to physically explore. To use Bruner's (1959) expression, the child who actively seeks such physical experience displays a coping rather than a defending disposition with respect to his encounters with his physical environment.

Item 8: Play behavior with, for example, blocks is purposive. Block play may serve many psychological functions for very young children. Of interest here, however, whether blocks or other play materials are involved, is whether the child is attempting to carry out some intent, some scheme. As building materials which allow maximum latitude to the builder, blocks lend themselves particularly well to the idiosyncratic purposes of young children. Whether the child is attempting to join them in a line, pile them vertically, or simply juxtapose two individual blocks, intention or purposiveness can readily be observed. The methodical construction play capabilities of most non-handicapped two-year-olds often must be taught to a child unaccustomed to manipulative, motoric play. At any rate, the natural competence in employing means-to-end reasoning cannot be taken for granted.

Item 9: Uses objects as tools in achieving own purposes (e.g., a stick as extention of arm, a chair to stand on). Important evidence of problem-solving capabilities is the young child's use of some object as a tool, a means of augmenting his own body. Just as tool-creating and tool-using propensities among primates and, apparently, among the ancestors of Homo sapiens offer rich insights concerning the relation of hand and mind in an evolutionary sense, so such behavior in very young children evidences prototypic problem-solving behavior of great adaptive significance.

Item 10: Enjoys new experiences. Inseparable from physical exploration is an interest in novelty. Although infants may persevere with a familiar play object or imitative sequence for long periods of time, satiation with such practice play usually makes the new toy or game of much interest. In Piaget's terms, repetition of the familiar and interest in the new can be related respectively to assimilation and accommodation, between which there is constant interplay in order for mental growth to proceed.

Item 11: Enjoys investigating a new toy. This item inquires about a specific manifestation of willingness to explore new and unfamiliar ground. What the child does, that is, how he actually explores and comes to know (in the Piagetian sense) the new toy, is of course always fruitful material for observation. Parents often are eager to see what an infant or toddler will do when presented a new toy on a birthday or other occasion.

Item 12: Will persevere in problem-solving with toys or puzzles. In a sense, perseverance on the part of a two-year-old with an age-appropriate task is quite comparable to the determination, achievement motivation, and need for closure which enables older children to experience academic success in school, master a musical instrument, learn to swim, or accomplish virtually any task which requires stick-to-it-iveness. Even for the toddler there is probably a conflict situation associated with a form board puzzle, for example, involving frustration and fear of failure on the one hand and the desire to complete the task on the other. Although adult approval is doubtless often a factor, the task itself may be sufficient to provide the motivation, as Maria Montessori believed. In Piaget's terms, the task must have an optimal level of difficulty: not so hard as to be overly frustrating, yet not so easy as to lack challenge or fail to amuse. J. McV. Hunt (1961) refers to those criteria for task selection for learners of any age as "the problem of the match."

Item 13: Reflects pattern in block building. Closely related to the child's purposive use of blocks is his mental awareness that they may be used to create replicas of objects or events in the world.

Block play thus provides an excellent indicator of the presence of representational thought, as well as creative ingenuity.

The third category of the Checklist, *Social Adaptation,* includes items relating to social adjustment in the group situation. Nursery school and kindergarten teachers have traditionally termed the behaviors involved in achieving such adjustment and socialization skills. The following items were included:

Item 1: Separates readily from mother. In light of the parent-child focus of Project HEED, all aspects of the child's behavior in relation to his mother were of great interest to staff. The ability of a child to separate at an age-appropriate point in his development may reflect awareness based on previous experience, that mother's leaving is not irrevocable; enjoyment of the nursery classroom milieu and feeling of safety and security within it; an attitude of trust toward the teacher as a temporary mother surrogate. Importantly, flat affect in response to initial separations in very young children may signal the presence of problems in object relations. First separation probably should, in most cases, be difficult for the child.

Item 2: Appears happy and content. The rating is based on subjective judgment made by the teacher. Explanatory comments provide substantiation.

Item 3: Shows awareness of peers as individuals. The emergence of awareness that people must be distinguished from inanimate objects is certainly noteworthy. The manner in which these children, many of whom have had no prior experience in associating with agemates, relate to their peers is observed carefully and is of great interest to the staff. The group dynamics of the classroom, including patterns of peer interaction, roles and friendships, are described in Chapter 10.

Item 4: Engages in parallel play. The development of social play usually proceeds from solitary (non-interactive) to parallel play behavior, to cooperative play activity. Preschool teachers commonly remark on the difference between the play of a two-year-old and that of a three-year-old. Obviously, there are many individual differences at every age level in play modes. However, parallel play is generally observed to appear in children exposed to opportunities for peer interaction during the third or fourth year. Blocks, as well as many other media, provide excellent opportunities for observation of children playing independently, yet in proximity and in relationship to one another.

Item 5: Can recognize the name of and correctly identify at least one peer. Knowledge that another child has a name, as he himself does, suggests that the child's social world is beginning to take some form. It is interesting to note which peer becomes especially significant to a child. This point is illustrated through descriptions of several examples in Chapter 10.

Item 6: Initiates interaction with peers. Awareness of peers is a necessary but not sufficient condition for cooperative social interaction. The interaction noted here will usually fall far short of cooperative play *per se,* that is, action performed collectively or in concert, but signals a prelude to such truly reciprocal cooperation.

Item 7: Initiates interaction with adult other than parent. The interaction may be with a staff member or mother-helper. The willingness and ability to relate to and to interact with an adult in the role of teacher suggests a degree of social maturity, confidence, and security in the classroom environment.

Item 8: Vocally refers to one or more peers as individuals. The child need not be able to execute an articulate or even accurate vocalization. If the child, however, has some vocal means which he employs with consistency to identify a peer, he is manifesting awareness of the individual identity of others.

Item 9: Will follow a simple verbal instruction. The questions are not, "Does the child always follow instructions?" and "Is he obedient to the requests of adults?" The psychological diagnostic assessment and that administered by the speech pathologist tap the child's ability to respond to verbal commands or instructions as an index of receptive language and association of auditory input with motor response. The question here is whether the behavior capability is present in the natural environment of the classroom.

Item 10: Joins in group activities such as singing, finger plays, rhythmics. These activities, so common to the usual experience

of three and four-year-old nursery school children, are introduced in the HEED classroom. The group participatory nature
of the activity is, for most of the children, a novel experience.
There is the opportunity for peer learning through imitation
and awareness of peers *qua* peers. A child's first response may
be to listen and look in apparent fascination. Attempts at participation are observed and encouraged.

Category IV of the *Teacher's Periodic Checklist* comprises a
variety of items relating to representational functioning and
concept acquisition. The following areas are assessed:

*Item 1: Engages in symbolic (representational) play (domestic theme,
transportation.)* The question here is whether the child's spontaneous play behavior is dramatic, in the sense of reenacting
social interactions or conveying themes. Imagination is promi-
nent in the spontaneous play behavior of most three-year-olds
and is a manifestation of assimilation as experiences are internally represented through the child's own mental structures.

Item 2: Vocally narrates own play. With or without words, representational thought is revealed through the play of children
who in some form narrate their activity. Pushing a toy car with
accompanying sounds, "Vroom, vroom," qualifies, although it
is not nearly so complex as the narratives which can be over-
heard as many three and four-year-olds play.

Item 3: Will imitate an adult behavior when directed.

Item 4: Will imitate an adult behavior spontaneously. The child
who will follow a teacher's (or other adult's) direction and
example in an act such as nose-touching or hand clapping is
demonstrating his ability to attend and to respond. Spontaneous imitative behavior shows more initiative on the part of the
child and interest in his social environment. Deferred imitation,
it is assumed, occurs developmentally later when a child may
recreate something observed or experienced long after the
event.

Item 5: Will imitate a peer behavior when asked by adult.

Item 6: Will imitate a peer behavior spontaneously. Imitation is
considered a fundamental and extremely critical learning
mode in young children. A major aspect of the rationale for a
group program for these very young handicapped children is

intended to permit relatively precise determination of patterns, trends, critical incidents, and the like. Such concerns relate to the following areas:

1. Duration, extent, and form of separation problems, and point in program when satisfactory separation was achieved.
2. Frequency, quality, and point of emergence of interaction with peers.
3. Frequency, quality, and point of emergence of interaction with adults (teacher, assistant, therapists, parents in classroom).
4. Frequency, form, and point of emergence of self-initiated motor activity.
5. Frequency, form, and point of emergence of imitative behavior.
6. Nature and extent of mother-child interaction.
7. Frequency, quality, and form of engagement in problem-solving.
8. Play level and form, preferred play materials, and mode of material use.

The task of completing the forms each day as soon as possible after the group session proved a demanding one, requiring absolute adherence to a daily regimen. Since during the first program phase each child was a member of a group which met twice weekly, the teacher was required to complete eight forms, that is, to document comprehensively the behavior of each of eight children following each session. The form certainly facilitated this process, yet fell short in terms of efficiency of a check-sheet or checklist mode of reporting. Here again, it was determined to take the option of more interpretive and at least somewhat open-ended reporting. Whereas quantitative indices are not only less time-consuming but yield data which appears more objective, the appearance of objectivity may be misleading. Since a lower premium was to be placed on manipulation of data than on team sharing of insights concerning each child as part of the on-going formative evaluation process, the form was intended to facilitate expression of such insights. On a continuum which could be called *Quantity of Information*

Conveyed, the *Teacher Daily Record* items would lie decidedly toward the pole near which would be located comprehensive daily logs, but doubtless required the sacrifice of some information in order both to specify precise foci and to permit a manageable task for the teacher.

Those team members directly involved on a daily basis with the children, the teacher, the teaching assistant, and the physical therapist describe the daily record, although extremely time-consuming, as a valuable device for bringing continuity to each child's experience. Looking at these observations concerning a child's accomplishments or other pertinent data, over a period of time, served to direct intervention efforts in a more planful manner than would have been the case if recollections had to be relied upon. As a communication means for other staff members to follow continuing progress of individual children in a most economical manner, the daily record proved invaluable. One of the principal users of these always "fresh" data, always immediately available in each child's folder, was the caseworker. Through regularly reviewing the record form, the caseworker was in an excellent position to share interpretations of a child's behavior with the parent, who might have many questions and concerns formed through observation and participation in the classroom activities.

In addition to the caseworker, who also found the forms helpful in the preparation of communications with referring and consulting pediatricians, orthopedists, and pediatric neurologists, the psychologist and those special therapists not involved daily with each child found the record forms useful. Without the on-going picture of the child's functioning in the natural setting of the classroom, prescriptions provided by these specialists to be carried out by those in daily contact with the children would be of limited value. Use of the daily records, together with weekly staff meetings, treatment staffings at three and six month intervals, and intentional provision of a built-in forum for informal communications, provided assurance of common ground whenever a child was discussed. One may often hear, in treatment or social agency dealing with children, therapists, teachers, or others describing what seems almost very much like two or more different children. Communication across disciplines is frequently ragged and sometimes absent altogether, and the distrust and even hostility existing between professionals representing different disciplines is notorious.

There can be little doubt that effective communication is the *sine qua non* of coordinated team effort on behalf of the child. Consequently, communication was from the outset given the highest possible priority by the HEED team.

THE ELEVEN O'CLOCK RAP SESSION

The informal communications vehicle alluded to earlier is not any the less vital for the looseness of its organization and format. Although teacher, physical therapist, and teaching assistant require considerable additional time in planning, the gathering of staff at the conclusion of each session for debriefing came to be regarded as indispensable. This period, usually lasting about one hour but often spilling over into the lunch hour, came to be known as the eleven o'clock Rap. There was never an agenda; attendance varied; no one led or directed the discussion which often ranged far afield, but the value of these highly enjoyable sessions soon became apparent to all concerned.

While putting away materials from the children's activities or sitting in the child-sized chairs or on the rug, participants in these discussions sometimes heatedly, often humorously, described occurrences, offered advice, and raised searching questions. This often became a forum for intense debates and for the airing of disagreements.

In addition to the teacher, physical therapist, and teaching assistant, regular participants were the project director, caseworker, physical therapy supervisor for the agency, occasionally joined by other team members. This unbroken communication link served constantly to relate understanding of the families and educational and therapeutic work with the child. Often, problems would arise requiring immediate planning, or information in need of prompt dissemination and response. The daily informal meetings provided a communications center for dealing with these needs.

The usual focus for discussion, however, was some new behavior observed either by a staff member who had been interacting with a child or by another who had been observing the interaction. Frequently, discussions concerned whether a child had, in fact, used a new word or more complex language structure and, if so, how the staff person involved had responded. In these instances, criticisms were offered freely and accepted without resentment. The discussion of what had occurred in a specific instance achieved closure with consensus regarding future planning and decisions to try out specific strategies.

The caseworker was often able to report a concern or question raised by a mother who had observed the session, and on many occasions an insightful observation or useful suggestion made by a parent. Conversely, staff observations concerning a mother's interaction with her own child and other children during the activity sessions usually provided new insights for the caseworker.

Discussions concerning problems in behavior management with specific children, as in the case of a boy who initially acted out in a hostile and destructive manner, may result in strategy decisions. In this instance it was determined that the teaching assistant would maintain a one-to-one relationship with Gerald at all times, both to prevent harm to other children and to Gerald himself, and to enable him to feel more secure in his new surroundings.

TEAM MEETINGS

Beyond the daily informal communications and constant staff use of record files, a regular formal structure is required for the dissemination of announcements, the sharing of views, and the detailed review of progress of each participating child and parent. A weekly team meeting serves this function, with all project personnel present.

The meeting is chaired by the Project Director, who follows an agenda comprising items raised during the preceding week by staff members. The agenda for each meeting is determined by whatever problems may have arisen during the week or may be looming for the immediate future. In addition to formal staff conferences on each child, meetings may deal with new entries to the program, scheduling concerns, and often special topics of interest, such as nutrition or other substantive areas, presented by a resource person.

These discussions are coordinated and mediated by the project director, who often finds it necessary to make final decisions regarding project policy or practice issues which arise. However, the structure is democratic and the expertise of each team member is respected and brought to bear in decision making.

Among their other functions, however, the team meetings served the vital and indispensable role of coordinating and directing the work of the team. Without the opportunity for all staff members in concert to review the progress of all children and thus to determine objectives and strategies, the concept of a team approach would be hollow.

The preceding discussion was intended to underscore the important role of communication among members of an interdisciplinary team. Although differing methods may be employed by individuals trained in various disciplines, the major questions they address are of significance to all and often relate to superordinate dimensions of the child's functioning, dimensions which transcend the scope of a specific discipline or approach.

Chapters 13 and 14 describe the application of the formative evaluative procedures employed, first within the framework of individual case studies and second in terms of their use in the determination of program effectiveness. The two chapters which follow deal directly with the role of parents of the handicapped child, first in terms of personal needs and interpersonal dynamics which must be considered, and second in the form of an analysis of the parent component of Project HEED.

CHAPTER 5

PARENTS AND THEIR
HANDICAPPED CHILDREN*

T HE ROLE OF PARENTS has always been regarded as crucial in
the growth and development of their children. In recent
years, the critical influence of parents has been noted at pro-
gressively earlier periods in the life of the child, including the
important influences of the child's intrauterine development.
This trend indeed has basis in the area of organically related
developmental problems, as many abnormalities, handicaps
and disease syndromes can be traced to genetic influences or
experiences during prenatal development.

The focus on the role of parents is particularly significant in
view of the marked change in the types of diagnoses accompanying referrals to a modern rehabilitation center. With advances in medical knowledge concerning disabilities and handicapping conditions, acquired illnesses like poliomyelitis, tuber-
culosis, or rheumatic heart disease no longer require as much
attention and service in a center for rehabilitation. Instead, an
increasing number of children with congenital ailments are
seen, problems which carry with them different manifestations
in physical handicapping conditions than those seen by such an
agency in the past. Typically, there are also differences in the
psychological reactions and expectations elicited by the condition, both in child and mother, as well as other family members.

In dealing with this basic area of the child's psychosocial
growth, the professional person must be aware of the many
factors that will influence the mother-child relationship and
how judgments might depend on one's own point of view and
the background against which observations of the interactions

---

*The authors are indebted to Ann S. Newman, Casework Supervisor of the Society
for Crippled Children of Cuyahoga County, who assumed major responsibility for the
preparation of this chapter.

SEPARATION AND DEPENDENCE

A mother's ambivalence or burden of self-blame may in many ways prevent her from fostering in her child the feelings of autonomy essential to his optimal development. Fearing that he may injure himself if allowed to explore on his own or that it is her duty as a good mother to attend to him at all times, she may instead foster in her child an undue and unnecessary dependency which is detrimental to his growth as a person.

A similar pattern of behavior can often be observed where mother and child seem to have difficulties in separating. If the situation is observed closely, it is usually quite obvious that it is the mother, rather than the child, who seems unready to make the separation. She may put many obstacles in the way of the child coming into a program. She seems to need the child to be dependent upon her and to act out for her the role of a child that cannot separate. With help, the mother may be able to face the separation, but frequently mothers with such needs as these will drop out of a program and seek other medical opinions and other medical devices for a solution to the child's problems.

Often, as is discussed further in a subsequent chapter, the mother may experience feelings of inadequacy or even unconscious resentment of the successes the professional therapists and teachers in an agency may have in areas in which she has been less successful. At times, a parent may find progress difficult to accept, and a child's gains may ironically precipitate a desire to terminate his participation in a program.

The problem of dependency as it relates to the adjustment of handicapped children, then, is a two-sided coin. Without conscious realization, a child's mother, or even both parents or an entire family, may become overly dependent on the handicapped child for fulfillment of needs. Just as certain parents of emotionally disturbed youngsters are thought by professionals to "need a sick child," and therefore to impede efforts to help the child, parents of a child with a physical handicap may quite unconsciously maintain patterns of interaction with their child which are inimical to his growth as an autonomous person. Such needs may stem from the substitute gratifications a mother or father may have derived in their caretaker roles. They may represent manifestations of feelings of guilt and a form of penance, even martyrdom. It is the task of the professional caseworker to help such parents discover more adaptive modes of coping, both in their own interests and in terms of the child's needs.

It is not uncommon for a guilt-ridden parent, or for one who is simply determined to be all to her handicapped child, to experience occasional or even simultaneous feelings of resentment toward the child or to project onto the child the intense self-hate from which she suffers. Such feelings may at times find overt expression. Whether angry impulses are acted upon and feelings of resentment, rejection, and hate are acted out in dealings with the child, they will probably color the parent-child relationship, and hence the child's self-feelings. In her effort to guard against these dangerous impulses and to counteract feelings of anger and rejection, the parent may become even more solicitous. Overprotection and oversolicitude, too, result in a form of deprivation for the child, whose strivings for independence and a sense of mastery are made even more difficult by the physical handicapping condition itself.

DENIAL AND ACCEPTANCE

When parental grief and guilt, most commonly on the part of the mother, go unresolved, as is often the case, care of the child and attending to the implementation of an appropriate medical, habilitative and educational program for him are far more difficult.

Often the mother will try to make herself more comfortable by denying or minimizing the degree of handicap or her own involvement in it. These denials take many forms, some of which are easily recognizable, but some are subtle. In the former group are those in which the achievements of the child are exaggerated. The mother says the child is toilet trained, for example, but the child comes in to the rehabilitation agency in diapers. There is the mother who readily accepts all suggestions but never quite succeeds in carrying them out, or the mother who insists that suggestions and programs will not work even before trying them. In this type of behavior, a mother may often say that there is no problem at all, so why carry out the program? Or she really does not want a solution and prefers simply to hope or believe that the problem will go away.

A more subtle form that such denials may take occurs when all suggestions and appointments appear to be carefully kept. However, somehow the mother never gets to the appointment on time, or things keep happening at home so that the child never arrives for treatment or the mother never gets an opportunity to do the program at home. Excuses run the gamut, including loss of car keys, a child vomiting while being dressed, and so forth. The list which could be cited is too long for elaboration here, but it is important to recognize and be able to deal effectively with such devices in behavior.

It may often be best to accept parental defenses such as these to get on with the business at hand, rather than to try "to work them through." Defenses are useful to an individual and, in dealing with parents of handicapped children, often much more is gained than lost by accepting the defenses employed by the parents. The situation can become more complicated if sometimes these defenses break down. This can occur, particularly, if the child does show more improvement than the mother seems to have been able to expect. The child can no longer provide for the mother the same form of satisfaction and, strange as it may appear to observers, the mother seems unable to accept the improvement.

Parents of physically handicapped children, like many parents of the retarded, may "shop" for a diagnosis which is easier to accept. Some personal experiences which frequently will color the interrelationship are tied in with guilt or shame. The idea of deserving punishment is frequently expressed by parents, such as parents who have been on drugs or who have a history of drinking. The big question is "What did I do to deserve this punishment?" And in spite of the fact that the community can and does accept more easily many individuals who deviate from the norm, there is often still a great deal of

shame experienced in having given birth to a handicapped
baby. With it is often an associated wish to undo and to have the
child reborn well and whole. There is also complicating the
situation the uncertainty of the baby's development and the
exact meaning of the doctor's diagnosis. There is resentment of
the caution that the doctor must show in terms of prognosis.
Mothers frequently become very suspicious, and often they will
change doctors. The doctor's position is also very uncomforta-
ble. No one likes to bear bad news, and he cannot, in fact, be
certain of what developments there will be. And the parents
will push for an answer. When will the child walk? How well will
he be able to learn? Not only can the doctor not predict in many
instances, but the human tendency to listen to what one wants
to hear may result in the doctor's being quoted very differently
from what he has actually stated. Disappointment and bitter-
ness may follow, and parents may blame the doctor for what
has not occurred.

In addition, there might often be confusion about the diagnosis and the prognosis. The doctor may predict that the child
will walk, but he will not be able to say how well the child will
walk or how much the deformity will affect his walking. When
the walking finally does come about, frequently the child will
appear for the first time much more handicapped than mother
had ever fantasied, as he lurches and staggers uncertainly.

The concern about mental ability is one that is frequently
associated with a physical handicap. The enormity of this concern may be due in large part to the nearly universal tendency,
at least in Western culture, to be affected by appearance. If the
child looks and acts awkwardly, he is likely to be labeled as
mentally defective, even though the mother has been told that
the child's intellectual ability is not impaired. If he looks dull,
the mother has to be reassured frequently, even when the child
appears to be succeeding in his learning experiences.

Involved here are not only the dynamics of the mother's
personal reactions and behavior as an individual but also the
cultural patterns of her environment. Physical imperfection is
likely to have an impact on anyone, the degree and form of
one's reaction varying for different individuals. What is seen as

an imperfection depends not only on one's own identification with the problem, but also on what one's community thinks about it. A brace looks very disabling to the person who is not accustomed to seeing one. Good learning ability may often be more important to middle and upper middle-class parents than to lower middle-class parents. Ethnic groups also have individual and different standards and reactions to disabilities. Specific family patterns also are part of the environment that carry weight in influencing the mothering the child may receive.

The variety of factors which may militate against a mother's ability to accept realistically the nature and ramifications of her child's physical handicap is nearly infinite. However, psychological acceptance is a necessary precondition for effective coping, realistic planning, and serving the best interests of the child.

The following excerpts from case records serve to illustrate the special problems faced by parents of physically handicapped children.

REACTIONS TO BIRTH OF A HANDICAPPED CHILD OF A DIABETIC MOTHER WHO HAD A GREAT DEAL OF DIFFICULTY IN KEEPING APPOINTMENTS

"Were you angry at having a handicapped child?" "No," she said, "I was angry with the doctor." The husband wanted a general practitioner but she thought she should have a specialist. She did not say why; she just thought it would be the thing to do. He failed to check her urine, and she had a temperature from uremic poisoning on the day of delivery. Delivery was very difficult because of the size of the child. She hated the doctor so much that she wanted to sue. Her husband discouraged this. Unknown to him, she consulted an attorney who advised that, while it was probable that there was some neglect, he would be unable to get expert testimony so she dropped the procedure. She then consulted a priest who tried to advise her to overcome her hate. She did not think she hated the doctor now but she still blamed him for what happened with Steve.

As she was about to leave, she mentioned her concern about Steve. He watches children playing ball and this weekend she was quite shaken up when he was playing with a football that had been given him by his uncle, and he started to talk about playing ball when he is able to walk. As she said this, she turned her back and commented that she wished this would come true. I suggested working on the program and hoping for ambulation as he grows older. I did agree, however, that we could not be too optimistic about the future until we saw how he would develop with therapy.

I tried to take mother back to a discussion about the father's feelings and the shock of having a handicapped child born to him. The mother admitted that it was dreadful. She herself had been very upset because she was told of her diabetes and the child being critically ill on the same day. She admits that the father had to bear the brunt of carrying through the program recommended by the doctor. She remained at _____Hospital and the baby was transferred to _____ Hospital. Father is less optimistic than she is about the child's development. They quarrel about this, but she thinks she is realistic. She knows he will never make a complete recovery and wants to do all that she can so that he will not be any more handicapped than necessary.

EXCERPTS FROM THE RECORD OF A CHILD WHOSE PARENTS COULD NEVER ACCEPT THE CHILD'S WEARING A BRACE OR SPLINT

After a diagnosis of brain damage had been made by the neurologist, the mother questioned the obstetrician who felt there was nothing about the birth that could account for the damage. When the child was seven months old, the pediatrician referred them to a neurologist since the right leg had weakness. However, mother had also noticed from birth that the right hand always remained clenched and the thumb tucked under as compared with the other hand which relaxed and opened. There might have been some damage at five and one-half weeks since the baby was very ill with a high fever and in a vaporizer tent. The mother later in the interview admitted that she resented her child very much at this time, and there is some guilt and confused feeling that if this illness caused brain damage, she was somewhat to blame. She was not well at the time of the child's illness and still tired from section birth.

The child was examined by another neurologist who felt "out on a limb" more than ever and whose diagnosis was guarded. He did refer the child to a physiatrist who wanted them to try a splint on the clenched hand to be worn day and night. The child was by then learning to walk and learning to pull herself up on furniture, and mother could see that the splint interfered with the child's movement. Consequently, she had only tried it for one month and then removed it. The mother reported that the doctor was not pleased when they returned and requested that they try it for two more months, but she could not. The mother admits that the hand is now relaxing a little more and most activities are with the left hand. Father is left-handed and mother is not certain of child's handedness.

Mother pointed out how relaxed the child's hands were in a picture taken when she was three days old. She was very ill at the age of five weeks and had a fever of 105 degrees. They noticed that the fist was tightly clenched at seven months, and the right foot was dragging at the age of thirteen months. There were no convulsions or tremors and the doctor would only say that there had been brain damage. They were puzzled as to what this meant. They are confident that she is not retarded. She is talking, not clearly, but they understand almost everything. They just cannot return to the hospital. They were unhappy with the diagnosis and they don't want to put her through any more tests.

The doctor did not urge that an encephalogram be taken because the father objected to it. He has had many such tests as he has a steel plate in his skull as the result of a World War II injury. He really has had a hard life. His own mother died when he was young and his father remarried when the two boys were in their early teens. Because he never warmed to his stepmother, he joined the Army to get away from home. He does not like his current job, and although he adores the children, he is somewhat rigid in discipline. For example, if they call out at night, he does not think his wife should go to them to comfort them. He thinks this is coddling. They used to have terrible arguments about discipline and several times he became so angry he put his wife out of the house, but they seem to be together on things more now.

Regarding her early life the mother stated that she hardly remembers anything about her mother and sisters and she didn't think any of them liked her very well. Her father loved and favored her but he died of pneumonia when she was twelve, and she then went to a foster home until she entered high school. "If I only had something to remember I might be a better mother," she stated. She knows she does not love her child enough in comparing herself to other young mothers who seem to have a confidence in handling their children that she does not feel. She would like family life to be "on a wonderful happy level" but knows it isn't that way.

The mother sat quietly while her husband took the initiative in this interview. He said he did not feel that the child had made much progress with the brace and he questioned its use, repeating what his wife had told us, that when the brace is worn the child is "rather listless and will not do anything." She will not perform on the toilet and will not play normally. Therefore, they feel that the brace should not be worn.

FAMILIES OF HANDICAPPED CHILDREN

An area which frequently does not receive attention commensurate with its importance is the role of the father. There appears today to be more interest in the father's role as a socializing influence in western culture than at any other time. This may, perhaps, be in large part due to the fact that family life itself is changing. Fathers are assuming a more important role in the rearing of a child in the traditional or nuclear family as well as in the experimentation and innovation that is being carried on with family life and modification of sex role stereotypes. Many fathers seem more ready and willing to assume responsibility for rearing the child and for caregiving than in the past. Even in the traditional type of family, the father's role is now recognized more realistically by professionals. The father who has wanted a son and then finds that he has a son who is handicapped may find it most difficult to adjust to his role, and his relationship with the child may as a consequence be very poor.

Feelings of frustration and grief are often very similar to those of the mothers but, because of strong cultural norms and prevailing societal attitude towards males, he has even less opportunity than the mother to express his grief and to be able to work through his feelings. In addition, regardless of the mother's status, he is the one who is usually out of the home and working; he may have fewer opportunities to become involved with the child and less effort is made by professionals to work with him.

As is the case with the father, not enough has been studied or explored about the siblings and their relationship to the handicapped baby. What few attempts have been made to uncover this area would indicate a great need for further exploration and study. It is rather interesting to note how frequently older sisters enter the helping professions, that is, careers that have direct bearing on raising or programming for a handicapped sibling, such as nursing, physical therapy, occupational therapy, social work, and special education. Often older siblings of a physically impaired child are observed to become very upset at seeing other handicapped children. Frequently a sibling will express great guilt or have nightmares which appear to be directly related to the handicapped brother or sister.

The mother's problem of dividing self between hospital and siblings at home was touched on earlier, but there is also the child that requires feeding every two hours, who sucks poorly, and who may take an hour for feeding. There are dressings to be changed for open ulcers; there may be a routine medication to follow. There is a postural drainage to do, and there are the ileo bags or diapers to change. Braces and corsets must be put on, or hearing aids protected from abuse, and in general home life can be disrupted, and often little approaching a satisfying family life can be established.

It must be remembered that no family is without stress. Feelings of anomie or frustration with one's career, conflicts experienced by women associated with fulfillment of the wife-mother role on the one hand and personal self-fulfillment on the other, inter-generational conflicts, and a variety of additional sources of stress may be latent or already manifest prior to the birth of the handicapped child. Thus, this event may activate or exacerbate problems in marital communication, child rearing, or other facets of family life not directly related to the addition to the family constellation of a handicapped baby.

The caseworker in an agency serving handicapped children works with a child's parents primarily around management of the child's physical and psychological needs, centering also on their own needs as parents of a handicapped child. Consequently, casework will tend to emphasize such areas as the implementation of a home program, the securing of rehabilitative services, and the formulation of future plans appropriate to the child's needs and capabilities. Some of the difficulties frequently experienced in enlisting the participation of parents in consistent and meaningful habilitation efforts have been described earlier.

Management of these problems present great challenges to those working in a program of rehabilitation of children, especially if parent-agency communications break down. However, it must be recognized that many times the apparent problems may cover up even deeper emotional conflicts and may represent the acting out of anxieties which often can be controlled only in what may appear to be a maladaptive manner. Staff frequently feels that results can be obtained through talking or counseling the parents in a directive manner. It is difficult not to push or to attempt to control. We are all drawn by the need to change things for the better and, if only unconsciously, fantasize ourselves as gods able to undo and to change the overwhelming problems that are presented in individual situations. Often, however, the reward of the professional must come in the knowledge that he has given his best by simply recognizing the genuine conflict experienced and by helping the parent to cope as effectively as possible.

CONCERNS AND FEARS FOR THE FUTURE

The major questions a parent of a handicapped child will have, although they may often be unspoken, pertain to what the future will hold for him. Parents, often on the basis of advice from professionals, relatives, or friends, will at times delay initiating therapeutic interventions in the hope that the difficulty will be outgrown. Even families who have access to appropriate clinic, agency, and special nursery school facilities when their child is young will experience legitimate anxiety as the time approaches when important decisions must be made concerning regular or special class or school placement, or even residential placement.

The parent program component of Project HEED, described in the next chapter, while addressing present realities in terms of parent needs and parent-child interaction, reflects the awareness of the professional staff that these parents are also, as they must be, oriented toward the future, toward what will follow the HEED experience. Consequently, the attempt is constantly made to assist HEED parents in their efforts to obtain information upon which realistic, appropriate, and satisfying planning may be based. On another plane, however, the need of parents to express their fears and to gain mutual support through sharing such concerns with others who face similar uncertainties, is recognized and respected.

CHAPTER 6

PARENTS IN THE PROGRAM: MODES OF HELPING*

To UNDERSTAND THE ROLE of the parents in the HEED program, it is important to see their experience as a gestalt as well as to examine the distinct forms of helping experiences in which they have participated. Parental participation in HEED occurs in a highly individual manner, as each parent listens, questions, watches, absorbs, discusses, rejects, is angered, feels hopeful, feels depressed, understands, fears, or is confused. Gradually, each individual has taken what is meaningful for her or for him from the variety of experiences available and the human contacts both with professionals and with other parents.

Once parents of a handicapped child come to a social agency, such as The Society for Crippled Children, they have already taken a step toward understanding and striving to meet the needs of their child. Participation in a program as demanding as HEED requires another major step, both realistic and difficult, in their perceptions of and responses to having a child who is handicapped. A parent will not enter, or certainly will not stay within a program such as this until he is able to share with others, if only by his very presence, a part of that painful experience.

Parents have come to HEED from all sections of the community, from all parts of what is called Greater Cleveland, which includes much of Cuyahoga County. Their racial, socioeconomic and educational backgrounds reflect the rich diversity of this cosmopolitan metropolis. In age, they range from late teens to early forties, and families with just one child and families with several seem to be equally represented.

---

*The authors are indebted to Marguerite Campbell, HEED caseworker, who assumed major responsibility for the preparation of this chapter.

concerned about. However, she may need to ask that one before she can get to what is really bothering her. Do you think
the child is retarded? Do you think he'll ever be able to go to
school? Will he ever walk? In HEED there is *time* for parents to
find the answers for themselves, to develop inner convictions
based on true understanding rather than on defenses against
guilt and fear.

The chasm between lay person and professional is narrowed
when parents come regularly to a program such as HEED. The
teacher is someone who is a person, rather than an authority
alone, as is the therapist, physical therapist, speech pathologist
and others. These are people whose hair looks better some days
than others, who sometimes feel enthusiastic and at other times
are tired, who may be absent because of a cold. They are people
and therefore easier for the mother to relate to. They don't
wear the mantle of professionalism that can be rather threatening and awe-inspiring to a mother. Instead they are almost
friends, people who know her child very well, can report to her
what he did in class today, and how he is doing in therapy.

Because there are constant encounters between the mother
and the staff, if she forgets to ask a question one day she can
always ask it the next time she comes in. A person with whom
one may exchange a recipe or share mutual discomfort over the
rainy weather is much less likely to be intimidating. In most
school situations when a mother is asked to come in for a
conference, she immediately assumes that her child has done
something wrong. If the child has a medical or psychological
problem, she may fear that she is going to be chastised for
something that she has done or has not done where the child is
concerned. In a setting such as HEED, where the staff is constantly accessible and where conversations between mother and
teacher and therapists take place in a very comfortable and
relaxed kind of setting, the mother is much less likely to be
tense and fearful and is therefore less defensive. Under these
circumstances the staff may also get new insight concerning the
parents. When one sees a mother twice a week and becomes
aware of the fact that she has another child at home who is ill or
who is having school problems, that she herself is not feeling

well, or that for the past few sessions she seems depressed, whether she says why she is depressed or not, one begins to realize that she has just so much time and energy to give to this handicapped child. Occasional failure to follow through at home on physical therapy routines or suggestions by the occupational therapist can therefore often be seen with greater understanding.

When parents remark on the advantage for the children of the warmth and attention of teacher or therapists, they also seem to be expressing their own discovery and satisfaction that others can find their children interesting and lovable. Indeed the attitudes of the staff, as well as their techniques, can provide a model for the parents which may be especially important because of the deep ambivalence that is common to parents of handicapped children. Staff attitudes toward the children, accompanied by their genuine understanding and respect for parents, can provide a healing balm for parents whose experiences have shattered their self-image and frequently made them very unsure of themselves. Staff members are informal and friendly and do not confine contacts with parents to professional discussions. Parents respond not only to the fact that each child's individuality and particular needs are recognized, but to the fact that they also are appreciated for themselves, independent of their children.

In such a setting with parents close at hand, professionals become personally aware of the problems and frustrations that parents may face in caring for their handicapped children at home. Their enhanced empathy for parents increases their ability to be helpful in responding to questions and feelings, offering suggestions and at times simply being good listeners.

Such proximity between professionals and parents also contains the potential for problems. In their close interaction with parents staff members relate as total human beings, with little opportunity to shield the less helpful aspects of their humanness, e.g. annoyance, prejudices, or over-identification behind a professional mask. Every staff member may not always feel either understanding or respect for every parent. Furthermore, with so many professionals involved, it is much more possible for parents to receive mixed messages or contradictory advice. There are several ways of dealing with such problems, which obviously require close cooperation between the disciplines involved. The social worker, who carries the chief responsibility for the parents' experience in HEED, often takes an active role in representing the needs of individual parents and the way in which they can best be approached by the staff. At after class rap sessions, as well as at weekly meetings, the professional workers frequently examine their own feelings as well as their professional thinking about the children, their relationship with the parents and the parents' individual needs.

When answering parents' questions, the staff makes a conscious effort to respond to parents in terms of the children's observed behavior in relation to their current stage of development and needs, rather than in terms of generalizations or labels. It is often possible to verbalize for parents the frustration, confusion, exasperation or other feelings behind a parent's question.

"I think I've pampered him." "Will she walk by June?" "I know you can't predict, but will he be able to go to school when he's five?" "You say he is able to chew, but it takes an hour to feed him already, and he just spits out the food on the table." The answers of staff members will vary, but usually they will contain some recognition of the parents' feelings. How hard it is to know what to expect of a child or what he is ready to learn when the parent's concern is naturally focused on his handicap. How difficult it is to live with the inevitable uncertainty about how the child will progress in the future. How exasperating the time-consuming daily care of a handicapped child can be.

In these informal contacts parents can and do exercise their own choice relative to which staff member they communicate with. This choice frequently reflects their personal comfort with a particular individual as well as the staff member's field of speciality. As parents struggle to understand and to deal constructively with their children's problems and their own feelings, they often use staff members to test their emerging thinking, particularly in relation to the degree of the child's disability and what they can expect of him. The opportunity to voice such feelings and thoughts to a sympathetic listener often precedes a parent's readiness to engage in a fuller discussion with the social worker. At other times it seems to provide parents with an alternative they prefer.

Each child entering HEED is given an initial evaluation by each of the disciplines involved—the teacher, the psychologist, the physical therapist, the speech pathologist, and the occupational therapist. The purpose of these evaluations is discussed in group meetings as well as in individual interviews with the social worker. Subsequent evaluations are scheduled at six month intervals. Parents are present during some of these evaluations and their own observations of what a child is doing are of importance to the staff. They are always given an opportunity to discuss the results with the professional involved if they wish.

In the long run these objective evaluations of the child's specific performance in various areas seem to be helpful tools in parents' growing understanding, acceptance and ability to handle their children appropriately. On the other hand, a parent who is new to the program can be both overwhelmed and threatened by having his child "looked over" by so many professionals. Already vulnerable, they may often feel that their ability as parents is being reflected in all these "tests." At a deeper psychological level, most parents have not yet come to feel and perceive their children's separateness from themselves. At this point the sensitivity of the professionals and their ability to convey respect and acceptance of parents are essential. The educational goal is to help each parent sharpen his own perception and understanding of a child's behavior in order that he may feel an enhanced confidence in his own ability to meet the child's needs.

DETERMINING THE PARENTS' ROLE

The HEED schedule for parents, that is how parents spend their time when they bring their children to the program, has evolved and changed during the first year in response to par-

comfortable observing from the observation room. When a mother observes from the observation room and a member of the staff explains and interprets to her what is going on in the classroom, she may be then better able to grasp what the program is about. Without the burden of anxiety about her role as co-teacher or feelings of inadequacy in her role, she may be therefore more attentive to what she sees happening in the classroom and to the explanation that is given.

THE PARENT GROUPS

Another important means of learning are the HEED group meetings which have included both discussion of topics raised by parents and also staff presentations on such subjects as physical therapy, speech therapy, the use of toys, and the development of a sense of self in children. Talks by professionals are always informal and planned to allow opportunity for group discussions and questions. Sometimes subjects raised by a specialist are discussed more thoroughly in the less structured meetings with the social worker.

For some parents the more unstructured meetings have provided a most welcome opportunity for mutual support and growing acceptance and understanding in the sharing of troubled feelings of anger, guilt, and frustration. A parent who is currently very overwhelmed by her situation, not necessarily just in relation to her handicapped child, is usually the catalyst for such an exchange. In such a case the challenge to the social worker is to extend such an opening of feelings to discussion which is meaningful for other group members, particularly in relation to the problems of having a handicapped child.

Other parents, less able to reveal as much of themselves, have nevertheless benefited from examining together how to handle their concern about subjects such as sleep, feeding, discipline, toilet training, relationships with doctors or the comments of strangers about their handicapped children. In such meetings the leader encourages parents to consider the feelings that underlie their handling of specific situations.

One or two of the parents have been openly hostile to the idea of attending any group meeting that was not organized around a more or less formal presentation. One mother announced at her first meeting that she had not come to the agency to join a "therapy group." Her negativism was more pronounced than that of other group members, but it struck a chord of response in several other parents who found the meetings to be too formal (i.e. making them feel tense as opposed to informal talking outside of meetings) or too frequent. Although there was less resistance among parents to meetings which featured presentations by a staff member, thus requiring less personal involvement, it became apparent that parents could also feel pressured by any presentation which in effect pointed up the disability of their children. Some parents seemed to need more breathing space to absorb the various services of HEED. Coming to grips with one's own child's disability is a painful process.

Both the attitudes of individual members and the chemistry of the groups have affected group meetings and how they have been handled by the worker. It has seemed important to encourage the expression of all feelings, including those about the group itself. For some groups it has seemed best to provide a more structured presentation to stimulate discussion, and it is often difficult to secure appropriate visual aids or other discussion material. Some reading matter is too difficult for some group members, and relevant films and tapes are hard to find. HEED has been fortunate to have available knowledgeable professionals at the sponsoring agency who have been willing and able to share their knowledge and experience at parent meetings. The parents' own experience in the observation room can also be a point of reference for the group. It may perhaps become possible to have as a speaker a parent who has "graduated" from HEED, who would be willing and able to discuss his or her experience in later years, a subject of anxious concern for many parents.

Group meetings have been periodically modified in various ways. At times they have been held less frequently and are no longer held more than once a week. About a month is allowed to intervene after a new group of parents join the program, usually in September and January, before starting group meetings, although the program has single new admissions and withdrawals sporadically throughout the year. In initial interviews with parents the social worker introduces some of the topics that seem most appropriate for discussion later on. Indivdual interviews can be used to advantage in preparing the way for meaningful group meetings. Despite the problem raised by group meetings, for the worker as well as some parents, the method has proven itself to be an appropriate and effective means of communication, with its own unique value for parents in the HEED setting.

A pot of coffee is the only support service offered for one of the most important parts of the HEED program, the parents' own informal relationships with each other. When group meetings are not going well or a distressed parent does not want any professional help, it is reassuring to remember that HEED has brought together a vital and effective network of mutual interest and support. For many mothers HEED provides an important social life that is sometimes not available to them any other time. The opportunity for gossip and laughter and talk about the late night movie can be as necessary for them as their shared confidence about their children, their families and their personal problems. Staff members who have a free moment frequently join them.

CASEWORK WITH PARENTS

Casework in HEED has to some extent been dictated by the amount of time available. Initial interviews have become more structured and have come to include more specific information about daily parenting, such as feeding, toileting, discipline, and the child's experiences with other children and adults, as well as parents' understanding of the child's diagnosis. This interview can frequently serve to point out areas of parental concern for the social worker or other staff members to consider with parents in the future. Later the social worker may counsel individual parents at their request or around problems that are brought to the worker's attention by HEED staff, or at times of crisis concerning medical or family problems. All parents are seen following six month evaluations in order to interpret these and provide parents an opportunity to discuss them. When children leave the HEED program, the social worker works with them in planning referral to appropriate programs.

Although the social worker does not have the time to see most parents individually on a regular basis, when she does have an office interview, she can draw on extensive knowledge of the parent's and child's experience in HEED. Usually she has some basis for knowing where the parent is in her thinking and what the child is doing in the classroom. This mutual knowledge often enables the parent and the worker to focus more quickly on problem areas. Office interviews may be used to discuss what is going on at home with a child, another situation at home that is distressing a parent, a parent's feelings of guilt and anger about having a handicapped child, or a parent's emerging thinking about how best to handle a problem situation. Often casework can serve most effectively to provide an opportunity for more private or more extensive consideration of problems that have been discussed at group meetings or raised in the classroom situation by other members of the staff. As HEED staff has become increasingly more involved in discussing child management advice as individual problems arise in the classroom, the worker has had more time to work with parents as they struggle to find their own answers to the questions of what is best for their children and themselves.

It is difficult to generalize about changes in parenting that come about through participation in HEED. However, several themes to which parents often respond within the first few months have become apparent. Frequently, they are stimulated to think about and reconsider what their handicapped children may in fact be able to do for themselves, whether it be moving around on their own rather than being carried, feeding themselves, or being given the opportunity to help others. Along with such thinking, for some parents, comes a willingness and ability to set more appropriate limits with firmness and conviction about the child's readiness for a new level of expectation.

For a few parents the problems are reversed, and their experience in HEED helps them to become less demanding about expectations that have been unrealistically high, as they acquire a better understanding of developmental levels and sequence or the ramifications of their child's handicap. Others respond particularly to suggestions regarding toys or activities which meet the current developmental needs of their children. A few show very little change in their functioning as parents, where often professionals would like to see some change, yet they may come regularly and express deep convictions about the importance of the program both to them and to their children. These differences in response reflect the depth and complexity of the parents' own feelings about their children and about themselves. Whatever therapy and whatever improvement in functioning and adjustment HEED can offer to these young children, now or in the future, their parents must still live with the painful fact that the children will remain handicapped forever.

CHAPTER 7

THE EARLY LEARNING ENVIRONMENT*

ROLE OF THE PHYSICAL SETTING

WHEN IT IS CONSIDERED in relation to the psychological development of human beings, the concept *environment* is often used in a highly abstract manner. In Piaget's theory, for example, continuous interaction with the environment is the necessary condition for the reciprocal processes of assimilation and accommodation. In much current writing on education, emphasis is placed increasingly on the importance of the environment in which learning occurs.

That the role of the environment in influencing behavior must be idiosyncratically determined is strongly implied in Kurt Lewin's famous formula, B = f(P,E) (behavior is a function of the person and the environment), where the last term is assumed to be a psychological environment. This suggests that forces in that environment are a part of the individual's psychological reality at any given moment; elements of the objective environment assumed to have certain properties comprise a necessary but not a sufficient condition for bringing about behavioral change.

This point may often be overlooked by those who design and equip classrooms. The technique of photographing nursery classrooms from the perspective of the user, the child of three or four, may reveal a very different "environment" from that perceived by the adult, as Gloria Small (1973) has shown.

What constitutes environment? Irrespective of more abstract conceptual issues concerning the role of environmental factors

---

*Laura Gregg, HEED teacher, provided many significant contributions to this chapter.

in influencing behavior change, the parameters of environment as a "field," some pragmatic aspects may be discussed. Educators are accustomed to speaking of a classroom environment as, for example, rich, responsive, structured, and the like. The point which may be overlooked is that classrooms need not and usually do not, in fact, provide a static or constant environment. The "objective," physical environment itself, may be subject to modification.

The HEED classroom provides a helpful illustration. Although a variety of activities may take place at any given time, each teaching session invariably comprises three time blocks during each of which activities with specific features take place. As the children are brought to the classroom by their parents, child and parent are greeted. The mother and staff member will usually take the opportunity to converse, to share information, or to make arrangements for a subsequent conference. The child, with a staff member, will select a toy with which to play or an area of the room to explore: the carpeted area includes a full-length wall mirror, a ground-level easel chalkboard and other items. Soon, a variety of manipulative toys, formboard puzzles, and the like are in use, with some children shifting attention from one to another, while others persevere in an activity, such as pouring sand (actually a mixture of uncooked rice and other ingredients) in the domestic play corner.

During this time, one's perception of the global environment suggests a bustling milieu of exploratory and manipulative play, several simultaneous one-to-one adult-child dyads, one or more children quietly (or noisily) practicing repetitively with a stacking toy or pounding toy, and occasionally two children engaged with the same materials, whose play behavior may be beginning to approach the parallel stage.

At an appropriate moment, the physical setting undergoes a remarkable change. With "It's clean up time," and the flashing light signal, toys and materials are stacked, re-assembled, and picked up, and children, with much conscious and intentionally explicit guidance from staff, carry or push materials to the storage cabinet. This change is immediately followed by the appearance of the wooden ladder slide, "tunnel," leather cushion cylinders, and a four-foot inflatable ball. A total restructuring of the environment has seemingly been effected.

The room is now a different room, designed for different activities. Both children and adults manifest new expectations concerning what will take place. David gleefully crawls for the tunnel, as Teresa helps the physical therapist move the slide into position. She will be first, and a queue of sorts forms behind her. One by one, several children experience a ride on the big ball, stomach down, feet held firmly by the adult, who bends legs at the knees and encourages the child to touch the floor with his hands on the forward roll.

After a time, with the appearance of signs of satiation and fatigue, the large muscle equipment is returned to its storage alcove in the room. Each child who is able to knee-walk retrieves a chair from a side of the room and pushes it to a central area, where the teacher and her assistant have arranged the low tables in semicircular fashion. Soon, the setting, with its concomitant set of mutual expectations, is one of common, teacher-directed, group experiences: songs, a finger-play, conversation, and snack.

Although with a new building expansion program in progress, new facilities for the HEED program were being planned which adhered to staff recommendations. During its first year of life, temporary quarters had to be found for the program. It is often the experience of individuals involved in recent years in programs for young children that physical space provisions are made by fiat. The ubiquitous church basement, for example, as a site for Project Head Start and day care, has frequently provided opportunity for staff persons to demonstrate their resourcefulness.

A room was found for the new HEED program which had previously been used as a volunteer work room, OT shop, and storage area. Upon clearing it out (which required all the imagination and tact staff could muster, since new locations had to be found for a vast array of diverse materials and activities) the professionals who would comprise the HEED team were amazed. What had at first appeared a hopelessly inadequate site, much too small, unattractive, and odd-shaped, now suggested the potential of becoming a learning environment.

At one end of the room, a short corridor-alcove led from the building's front lobby to the classroom door, quite serendipitously suggesting a potential function as an area for one-to-one work with children, staff, and mother and assistance with wraps, impromptu conferences, and possibly even individual speech work. At the opposite end another alcove, this one within the room, led to a door which became the usual means of entrance and exit of mothers and staff who wished to be unobtrusive. A special feature of this portion of the room was a large office, which could be entered from the alcove, and which looked on what was to become the classroom through slightly tinted glass from slightly below waist-level to the ceiling.

While one would not expect a storage area to serve as a suitable environment for the handicapped child, the HEED classroom has proven more than adequate.

The physical smallness of the dimly lit corridor leading to the classroom provides a feeling of intimacy for children who are only two years old. This entrance way elicits positive anticipation for what might occur within the classroom. The sign, "Please knock, small children at work," is a direct invitation for the mothers, along with their children, to come inside. It appears that the child's attention gravitates toward the warmth and security of a bright shag rug located in a quiet corner of the room. Perhaps it is the combination of the texture, the color and the placement in the room that especially draws new children to this spot. Not only is it appealing to the newcomers, but the restless child usually responds positively. Many children seem to enjoy this area for story time or investigating books on their own. This seems to be the ideal spot for a small doll crib with assorted dolls that the children enjoy cuddling. A wall space problem necessitated placing a long mirror in this corner; however, it has proven to be a most important addition. Invariably, a small child can be found there viewing himself and studying his action, seeming to question his own image. Frequently, a staff member will place a child in front of the mirror helping him in self-discovery.

To the left of the door are three large windows that look into an office which is now being used as an observation room for parents and staff. The windows are set up about twenty-four inches from the floor and conveniently have a four inch ledge which the children can, and do, use to pull themselves up and wave to the adults on the other side of the windows. The child who recently experienced separation seems to derive comfort at seeing her mother on the other side. At one point it was suggested that a one-way mirror be installed to replace the clear windows. Since it was found that the presence of the parents for the most part is not distracting but comforting, the windows are now viewed as a positive addition to the room.

To the right of the door there is a long wooden counter with a small metal sink and yellow cupboards below. The counter is three feet from the floor, therefore not accessible to the children. The counter serves as a desk for the staff. During program sessions, videotape recording equipment is also kept on the counter, handy and ready for use. It is also used to mix paint or play-dough and to prepare the snack of the day and it is often used as a place to seat a child to be washed when he is covered from head to toe with paint. The cupboards below are used for storing dry clothes, cups and bowls for snack and musical instruments which the children are free to take out at any time.

Directly across the room from the counter on the west wall are floor-to-ceiling windows. They bring to the room brightness on even the dullest day. They provide the children and staff with a sense of the world outdoors. It is not uncommon for a child to crawl over to the window to touch and discover the smooth, cold surface or to view the everyday sights of sky, birds, trees, people, cars and trucks.

This entirely windowed wall proved a factor which lent a cheery and non-institutional touch. The view provided was that of a tree-lined residential boulevard, much trafficked by cars and trucks. The environment was thus enriched by visual access to the out-of-doors, but the degree of visual stimulation could also be regulated effectively through the use of attractive drapes.

HEED children from the outset appeared to have greater

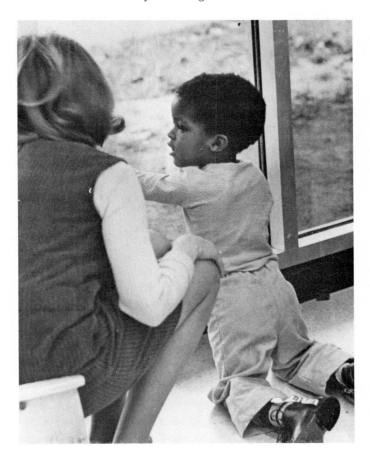

ability to monitor visual stimulation than is often seen among older brain-injured youngsters. Whereas the staff has often become aware, through videotape playbacks, that auditory stimulation, generated primarily by the many adults who may be simultaneously talking with children, has reached the level of noise, seldom does a child appear to be experiencing overload through the visual modality. One of the early HEED participants, an ambulatory child with cerebral palsy and considerable consequent brain damage, did appear overstimulated and manifested considerable non-directive activity. He appeared to require a much more restricted and bland environment.

However, it was surprising to note how readily the children adapted to the sight of anywhere from three to nine adults through the glass of what soon became an observation room. Occasionally, a child would glance toward the row of faces and exchange hand waves or smiles with a familiar adult, possibly his mother. Seldom did the sight of a mother reactivate anxieties over separation; on the contrary, the arrangement seemed made to order for reassuring both the child and the mother who might be experiencing difficulties with separation. The excitement that accompanies observations of interesting events outdoors often brings about spontaneous words such as *bird* or *car*. Such occurrences, of course, provide considerable excitement for the staff as well.

The white tile floor is very practical for gross motor activities such as toddler cars, tires on casters, standing and crawling activities and pull toys. It is also easy to clean after spilled paint or even an occasional leaking diaper. A variety of textures can be experienced by the children as they move from the coarse rug surface to the smooth tile floor. The soft white and yellow of the walls easily blends and remains in the background neither bombarding nor distracting the children.

Adjacent to the windows are two small tables. Placed on one is a large plastic basin filled with uncooked rice, dried split peas and alphabet noodles. On the other is a small wooden toy stove. Since this area is not centrally located it requires a great deal of physical effort on the part of the children first to crawl to, and then to pull themselves up to the table in order to begin to play. Yet it is a very popular play area and evidently worth the physical exertion. At times the children use this area to escape the activity that is taking place in the center of the room. The mixture is stimulating to touch, sound and sight. As the children take on a relaxed mood, they seem more free in vocalizing. Often the children engage in socio-dramatic play as they cook breakfast for a doll they brought along with them.

The importance of a hard, uncarpeted floor in working with young orthopedically handicapped children is well known. The tile surface facilitates standing and walking balance, and even crawling or scooting are enhanced, primarily through the feedback the child receives from his movements.

For some children, the hard surface may be hazardous if balance is uncertain. Many large motor activities, riding wheeled vehicles, in particular, as well as standing with table support in a play area may make falling likely. Occasionally, a child must wear a helmet, rather than inhibit his activity. Most professionals agree that the importance of working with these children on a hard floor surface, despite the discomfort for staff and the need for vigilance concerning child safety, far outweighs these disadvantages and must be considered "non-negotiable."

The value of a tile or similar floor surface is further demonstrated when children are told, "It's clean-up time," a singing activity in which most children learn to participate. Children take turns, with help from the teacher, in blinking the classroom lights. (This requires standing on a chair to reach the switch, with support from teacher.) The lights and song signal children to pick up and put away toys, shoving items across the smooth surface toward the storage cabinet. Later, each child can push his own chair toward the snack table.

There is a large semi-circular table that is directly below the observation windows. The table is used for a variety of activities. At the beginning of the session the chairs are removed and four select toys are placed on the table. This particular time has been the source of a great deal of interaction. Children stand next to each other with a toy in front of them. In no time one or all of the children are interested in the toy one of their peers is investigating. Before too long screams can be heard and a child is protecting his property from an aggressive peer. Playful teasing and non-intelligible chatter are not uncommon at this time. When paper and paint or clay and cookie cutters are the main attraction and the children are seated, the entire mood is changed. The children are more reserved and interact entirely with the media and utensils they are working with. Perhaps being seated accounts for this change or the activity itself is demanding their full attention.

The next activity is singing and finger play. While the teacher leads the singing the children observe or try to imitate sounds and motions. Once the children become familiar with a particular song they anticipate the teacher's movements. They seem to enjoy repeating the sequences. Everyone seems to know that snack time has at last arrived. This is a quiet time because while the children enjoy snack time, it is really hard work for many of them because of their various physical involvements. Once snack time is over the children know that their mothers will be coming to take them home.

LEARNING CENTERS AND ACTIVITY AREAS

Several areas of the classroom, then, are associated with specific forms of activity. There is a general parallel here to the learning center concept used in nurseries and kindergartens, and in the English Infant School. There is no play house; however, the housekeeping area and several other activities areas elicit a degree of fantasy play. A block area is integrated in its use with other small muscle play materials. Two forms of blocks are used: multiform wooden blocks and large cardboard brick blocks. Neither tends to elicit a significant amount of spontaneous use, although from time to time a child will spontaneously incorporate a small number of blocks in problem solving, perhaps, to sit or stand on while playing or reaching.

Children's utilization of the learning area concept contrasts markedly with that of older peers in the agency's nursery school programs. These children, ranging from mature three to five-year-olds, accommodate well both to the relatively considerable expanse of classroom space and to the learning center areas designated in discrete locations. These include an elevated play platform, with stairs; a story and music center; dramatic play area, with dolls and dress up clothes; a center for creative projects, and adequate designated spaces for gross motor activities, such as eurythmics and wheeled vehicles, and for small motor play (on counter and floor, at one side of the room).

Perhaps both the more limited motility and the smaller size of the younger HEED children suggest that optimal room size should be quite smaller, and room arrangement much less complex. Group size, too, is approximately 50 percent that of the nursery school groups. The HEED classroom is sufficiently compact so that even the most severely handicapped children can traverse its length. The children can, in addition, be aware of events in any area of the room. Also, the gross motor expressive needs are considerably less than for older children, although outdoor playground activities in the nice weather are extremely popular.

On the playground, HEED children may even share the area with nursery school youngsters. They enjoy being pulled in a wagon, playing with sand and water, climbing the much larger slide and descending with an adult's help. Some have been able to learn to ride a tricycle. When inclement weather precludes outdoor play, wheeled vehicle use can and does extend beyond the classroom when indicated, moving out into the corridors. Walking practice and stair climbing involve moving out of the classroom with the physical therapist or other staff member.

For the small group speech therapy sessions, it appeared desirable to isolate temporarily an area of the room in such a way as to screen out extraneous visual stimulation. A two-section plywood partition was constructed for this purpose. Each section is made up of four by eight foot one-quarter inch plywood sheets nailed to a frame. Each section can then be mounted on especially constructed slotted base pieces, one at each end. The sections can be easily slid into place, bases and all and moved about to any location. In addition, the sections can be lifted out of their bases and laid flat on the floor for specific purposes, such as ascent-descent practice with a low elevation or simply to introduce an element of novelty in the setting. The sections can be repeatedly painted by the children and can also serve as ad hoc bulletin boards for display purposes. When not in use, they are easily stored by being moved quickly to one side of the room.

USES OF TIME AND SPACE

Two of the most basic and general dimensions of human experience, time and space, must be seen as interrelated dimensions of a learning environment. Both comprise wide ranges of options to be considered and used selectively by the adults involved. Both also comprise areas of most important cognitive learning for young children, as will be discussed and illustrated in subsequent chapters. Children in the early years of life come to impose their own mental structures upon experience in terms of these areas of time and space, as well as other important, and related, areas such as causality.

Logistical decisions, such as decisions concerning what to do when and where, although often made intuitively, involve weighing insights concerning the child and his readiness against a set of objectives. An array of possible activities, together with the general dimensions of time and space, constitute the range of possible decisions. The duration of an activity, its temporal relationship to what has come before and what will follow, the sort of surface required for its implementation, the degree of extraneous stimulation which can be tolerated, the need for proximity to certain items, and a host of other considerations will determine where and when it will be undertaken with a specific child. Adults who work with young children can learn to employ these dimensions as aids in planning and execution, rather than to regard them as constraints and barriers against which one must work and for which one must compensate. The basic arrangement of a learning environment and the determination of a general schedule reflect such an appreciation of space and time, as does a willingness to modify and adapt flexibly when the need is present.

LEARNING MATERIALS

Parents, as well as professional educators, have in recent years come to be increasingly aware of the importance of manipulative play as a major modality by which infants and young children construct knowledge and integrate experience. Consequently, much attention has been directed toward the attributes of toys and other play materials. Parents, and educational program developers, as a consequence, have come to be highly receptive to the vast numbers of "educational toys" which have become commercially available in response to the recent awareness of the importance of early learning. As their means permit, adults seek to acquire the best materials available in order to guarantee optimal learning opportunities for their own young children or those enrolled in their program.

That many such materials are of great value and have been developed on the basis of accurate knowledge of child development is unquestionable. However, parents and teachers may often lose sight of the value of learning resources readily available in the home, resources traditionally used in the exploratory play of young children. Pots and pans, graduated plastic mixing bowls, brightly labeled food boxes, spoons of various sizes and shapes, may incorporate in many instances the same concepts as those contained in expensive toys, and may often have greater motivational value as children begin to imitate mother or seek to work along with her. Many such items can also be used to good advantage in a classroom situation, along with other items, and have the value of conveying to observing and participating mothers ideas of how they may be made available at home. Similarly, the perennial fascination of sand and water for children, when viewed in conjunction with Piagetian insights concerning the style and form of young children's cognitive learning, suggests the value of these media for children's use in both home and classroom.

The mixture of uncooked rice, alphabet noodles, and dried split peas used in the HEED classroom in lieu of sand is less likely to get in between braces and skin, causing painful chafing. In addition, however, it is observed to be in some ways superior to sand, offering as it does visual and tactile variety. Such mixtures of things to be poured and scooped, ultimately to be measured and compared, can be made from diverse ingredients and used by young children in myriad ways which elicit their curiosity and creativity.

In the HEED classroom, attention is given to each item selected for incorporation, since it is not considered desirable to crowd the area with a great many materials which may then be unable to be used to best advantage. Importantly, too, the environment must be kept manageable from the standpoint of the child. Consequently, items are considered in terms of their learning properties and the appropriateness of these for the children's developmental levels and in terms of their observed interests and preferences. Also, as was noted earlier, an important consideration is the learning benefits which may accrue to mothers who are observing and working in the classroom. Materials which are simple, inexpensive, and readily available are used whenever possible in order to model activities which may readily be carried over to the home.

In order to follow up on parents' interests concerning materials use, a toy library was established midway through the project. In addition to parental guidance materials, such as pam-

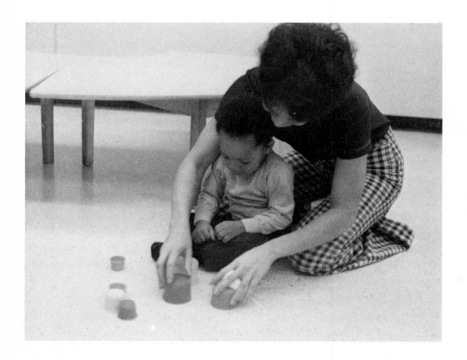

phlets, booklets, and even books, parents may also check out toys, puzzles, or other items, and mutual discussions among parents and those involving staff often are directed, as a consequence, toward developmental play and materials which will further its progress.

Although materials in the classroom may vary, depending upon the emergence of new interests and the satiation of old ones, and upon a certain amount of trial and error on the part of staff, the following items are normally in use:

Gross Motor

1 stuffed floor rocking horse (cushion-like)
1 Playskool® work bench w/tools
2 tires mounted on casters
2 dozen blocks (which open on the diagonal) 2" x 2"
8 large corrugated cardboard blocks
2 dozen wooden blocks 2" x 6"
1 large bag of assorted blocks—wooden and plastic
1 spring mounted rocking horse
1 small wooden sliding board
1 large bead arch
1 inflatable physical therapy ball—3′ diam.
3 rubber balls (1 small, 1 medium, 1 large)

1 Creative Coaster®
1 ATV® Explorer
1 pull train
2 jack-in-the-box
1 bee pull toy
1 helicopter
1 car and clown
1 Cry Baby Bear®
1 Jolly Jumping Jack®
1 dog pull toy
1 musical pull bear
1 Goldilocks and the 3 bears, playhouse w/people
1 Chatter® phone
1 milk wagon w/carrier and 6 bottles
1 pull toy lacing shoe
2 sets pop beads
1 tractor (riding car)
1 open-ended barrel

Fine Muscle Control

1 Dapper Dan® dressing doll
3 peg boards (2 wooden, 1 rubber)

2 boxes pegs (1 large pegs, 1 small pegs)
1 musical jack-in-the-box

Eye-Hand Coordination

3 larger wooden puzzles w/knobs (1 duck, 1 flower, 1 fish)
9 small wooden puzzles
2 small wooden puzzles w/knobs
1 Surprise Box®
1 wooden peg puzzle
2 form boxes (1 plastic, 1 wooden)

1 mailbox
1 stacking disc set
3 wire spindle and discs
1 threading block
1 nesting eggs set
1 nesting cups set
1 set nesting boxes (4)

Water Play

2 round rubber dishpans
1 large plastic boat (4' long)
4 terrycloth mitts

8 plastic aprons
assorted size plastic bottles and cups

Art Supplies

4 cans tempera paint
5 jars finger paint
4 long handle brushes
4 sponge brushes
4 paste brushes
1 large jar paste

4 boxes large crayons
15 paint pans (assorted sizes)
8 terrycloth smocks
assorted sizes and textures of paper

This procedure took a very long time and often seemed unsuccessful.

Since the advent of facilitation techniques of Bobath, Knott, Brunnestrom and Rood, prime importance is given to function. Although each proponent has her own specific theory concerning abnormal reflex patterns, each advocates total functional movement of joints. From the very beginning of therapy the therapist looks at the child as an integral person and works toward functional patterns of movement rather than the development of individual muscles.

A child's physical status must be elevated before goals can be set. A knowledge of reflex activity in children and physical development from infancy to full growth enables the therapist to plan a treatment program that is in keeping with the child's present status (Semans, 1967). Abnormal reflex activity must be eliminated or at least diminished enough to enable the child to overcome its action (Fiorentino, 1973). Although the ultimate goal is maximum function and independence, short-term goals are consistent with the present developmental level (Semans,

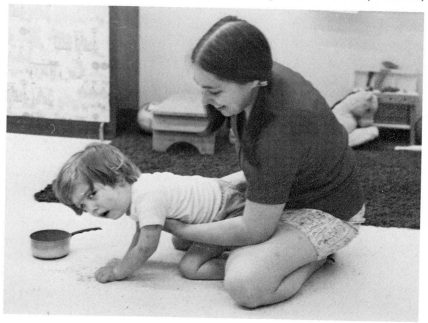

1967). Because immediate goals which are set too high produce frustration with ultimate refusal to accept further therapy, each session must contain activities which allow the child to experience some degree of success (Semans, 1967).

In a group program designed to increase motor function along with other areas of development, such as cognitive and communicative skills, the role of the physical therapist is still of importance. The therapist can encourage the very young child to participate in the program by positioning him so that he can work with the materials presented. It is important, however, to remember that each child must be treated at his own level of development regardless of what others in the group are accomplishing. This holds true whether the therapist is working on a one-to-one basis or is teaching gross motor activities to a group.

EDUCATION WITH THERAPY

In a rehabilitation setting most of the therapy is a learning-teaching situation. The patient must learn how to put on his own appliances and how to care for them. Patients learn a gait pattern; they learn self-care activities with the therapist teaching techniques that make accomplishing the activities easier for the handicapped individual. The therapy situation is really an educational setting with demonstrations, explanations, and problem solving of body management and activities of daily living by the patient and therapist together.

When treating a very young child, the therapist uses auditory, tactile and visual clues as well as proprioceptive stimuli to obtain the desired responses (Stockmeyer, 1967). A play situation which requires the desired activity provides the most meaningful learning and therapy for the child. The therapist adapts materials and work positions to each child's developmental level. To induce Keith to grasp, for example, his hands were tapped with a ring of keys and the therapist said, "Get the keys."

It is often necessary to reduce a functional activity to its simplest form. When attempting to teach a child to seat himself at the table, the therapist encourages him to push the chair to the table, keep one hand on the chair and the other on the table for balance. As he lowers his body to the chair, both hands are placed on the arms of the chair. When he is seated, he holds the edge of the table with both hands and pulls himself and the chair to the table.

An early education program, such as HEED, is an ideal setting for the very young handicapped child to learn cognitive skills along with motor skills. To encourage bilateral hand activities, the therapist may utilize a form box. The child uses one hand to pick up blocks and drop them into the slot while the other stabilizes the box. Simple puzzles consisting of two or three pieces with knobs attached enhance the therapy session because they are colorful and the finished picture brings satisfaction to the child. The child who needs to learn standing balance can complete the puzzle as he stands at a table which is the right height. Or, if the goal is to improve hip stability, the child may kneel at a low work bench to paint a picture. Sitting on the floor to play with a xylophone provides practice in attaining balance as well as the joy of creating musical sounds.

Keith needed to get up on his knees but he wasn't yet able to maintain the quadruped position. The therapist placed a bolster under Keith's torso with his knees flexed. This aided scapular and hip stability as well as enabling him to use his hands and arms to play with the materials the teacher provided (Finnie, 1970). It also gave him a different view of the world than he had had from a prone position.

An early intervention program which gives consideration to the child's motoric needs enriches the child's total experience and makes obvious the fact that therapy goals and educational goals are really inseparable.

THE TEACHING TEAM:
TEACHER, PHYSICAL THERAPIST AND
TEACHER'S ASSISTANT

The teacher, her assistant and the physical therapist, combining their experience and skills, can promote an environment rich in opportunities for the handicapped child to explore and develop. It is, therefore, imperative that the physical therapist working in a program such as HEED be thoroughly versed in the basic principles of early development, enjoy working and associating with very young children and be ingenious in the use of materials appropriate to the children. Because she acts as teacher and role model to the rest of the team, they become more effective in carrying out the therapy goals for the individual child.

After a child is evaluated and goals are determined, each team member is involved in administering the prescribed treatment. If the therapist has formulated an immediate goal of sitting balance on the floor for a child, the teacher encourages that child to spend portions of his play time sitting in the recommended position. When the teacher feels that a child is ready for the challenge of more complex materials, the physical therapist incorporates those materials into her therapy sessions.

Because each team member learns from the others, the physical therapist must be willing to explain and demonstrate her techniques to the other members of the teaching team. There are some undesirable positions that are assumed by handicapped children. The whole staff must work toward eradicating these positions and instilling the correct positions into the daily routine.

Sitting between the legs in a position commonly used by spastic cerebral palsied children. They assume this posture because it is easier than straight leg sitting. It gives them better sitting balance and allows them to play in an uninterrupted manner. Spasticity in some of the muscles does not allow for straight leg sitting but the easier position causes abnormal stresses on some of the joints and hinders good walking later on. Through the combined efforts of the adults in the classroom, improved sitting balance can be accomplished. It is the responsibility of the physical therapist to explain to the teacher and the teacher's assistant the need for proper sitting and positioning and how best to attain this benefit.

While working with play materials on the floor, the child may sit between his legs with the feet pointing out. The teacher, impressed with the child's concentration on problem solving, might overlook his improper position. The physical therapist might notice only the need for correcting his sitting position and ignore the fact that he is totally involved in a problem solving experience. As a team both therapist and teacher work toward appropriate goals without disregarding other areas of development. The teacher can ascertain that the child was in a correct sitting position when she first introduced him to the materials, or the physical therapist can quietly correct the posture without distracting the child from the task.

Many handicapped children do not like to be manipulated by teachers or therapists or even their own mothers. A basis for such aversion to tactile stimulation has been described by Ayres (1972) who has theorized an underlying tactile defensiveness. Chuck recoiled from staff members when he first entered the program. Even if he surmised that an adult might touch him, he pulled away. To attempt direct physical therapy with him at that time would have served no purpose. Instead, the therapist made no attempt to touch him but talked with him and played with him using the small cars which he loved. To build rapport with Chuck she incorporated the therapy treatments in play segments. They played catch to enhance standing balance and knee walked while pushing a chair, to improve hip stability. Within the classroom setting Chuck accepted her as a friendly adult playmate.

To attain certain functional skills children need to be encouraged into positions that are unfamiliar to them. Many do not like to be placed in the prone position because they are not accustomed to it. When placed on their stomachs, they attempt to turn onto their backs, or they may cry. Being part of a group can make it easier for the child to accept the new position because there are other children to watch, many adults to work with and interesting toys to play with. To secure the cooperation of the teacher, the physical therapist must make her aware of the importance of the prone position as the beginning of locomotion.

Peter enjoyed a sitting position because it was comfortable for him and he was familiar with it. When the physical therapist placed him on his stomach, he whimpered. The teacher quickly placed his favorite play material, the rice mixture, just beyond his reach and he attempted to reach it. With his attention riveted to the container of rice, he stretched his arms and trunk until he was able to grasp it and then played with it for a few minutes before he remembered his distress. Each session he remained on his stomach a few minutes longer until that position became comfortable and familiar to him. Gradually, he was able to pull himself along the floor on his elbows for short distances, and after several months his locomotion improved and he was able to reach toys he wanted or to get to the table for snack time.

EXPANDING THE THERAPY ENVIRONMENT

When the weather permits, the class is held outdoors. A large slide, wagon, tricycles and pull toys provide a variety of large muscle play experiences. Sitting or lying on the grass is a new experience for many of the severely involved children.

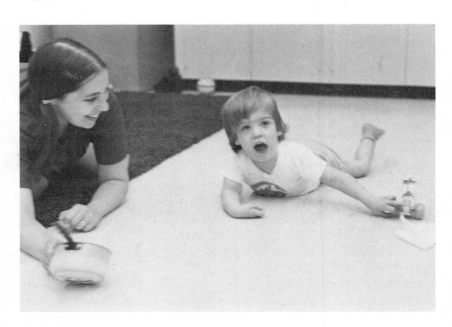

Although initially some of the children exhibited fear of the new surroundings, they all responded to the combination of fresh air, sunshine and play equipment. The patio provides a firm surface for riding tricycles and cars; the grassy area is fun for sitting, crawling and walking. The physical therapist, teacher and teacher's assistant are busy during outdoor play helping children climb up the steps and come down the slide, encouraging independent ambulation, or rolling a ball. Many handicapped children are denied opportunities for outdoor play so this provides them with another area to explore and additional motivation for motor development.

Cookies and milk, which are served at snack time, are stored in a kitchen down the hall from the classroom. When the teacher's assistant goes for them, she is always accompanied by a child who delights in helping to bring back a bag of cookies. His mode of ambulation is determined by the physical therapist.

A child who is walking with one hand support often accompanies the therapist on a walk to the secretary's office or to the nursery school as part of the therapy session. Purposeful activity and a destination add fun and excitement to a therapeutic treatment and give it additional meaning for the child.

Although eight children are enrolled in each HEED session, every child has his own program for developing functional motor skills, and the physical therapist carries the responsibility for incorporating appropriate therapy techniques into the child's total treatment program. Because the physical therapist views the classroom activities as aids to motor development for all the children, she actually implements two hour therapeutic sessions for every child.

ACTIVITIES TO FACILITATE LOCOMOTION AND ENHANCE GROSS MOTOR SKILLS

Children develop in a sequential order (Stockmeyer, 1967). A baby learns to hold his head up before he learns to turn over. He learns to crawl before he learns to walk. A child does not learn to walk and then go on to crawling, although some mothers point out that their child never crawled. If, indeed, a child should start crawling after he has been walking, he already knows how to crawl and need not learn to crawl at that point in time (McGraw, 1963).

With handicapped children there are deviations in the sequential progression. The child who is moderately involved in all extremities is encouraged to use the arms to pull himself along the floor. Many normal babies do this to move around their cribs. Babies pivot on their stomachs and with the use of their arms move themselves from one place to another. This activity is utilized with the handicapped child as the first means of locomotion. It sometimes entails going through the entire process of moving the arms forward, stimulating the muscles which must be used to pull and then gently pulling the child forward. This may have to be repeated several times before the child is able to manage without assistance.

When children are placed on the floor on their stomachs with interesting toys a very short distance away, the toys are often enticement enough for the child to begin moving on his own (Page, 1967). Once the child has reached the desired object, he is allowed to play with it. It is unfair to tease the child by constantly moving the object out of his reach just to keep him moving. The success of attaining his goal is important to him.

Pulling oneself along the floor on one's stomach is a primitive form of locomotion. As spasticity decreases in the lower extremities, the legs begin to assist in the pushing forward motion. When the arms are used to pull oneself along, the legs assist by pushing and, as the child's function improves, he learns to maintain the crawling pattern and then learns to move along in proper form.

If the child can stand and use his arms for support, he can push a cart or walker-type apparatus to get himself from place to place. Pushing a small chair can be an excellent means of locomotion (Finnie, 1970) which also enables the child to carry his play things from one location to another. At snack time all of the HEED children choose a chair and push it to the table.

For the child who cannot ambulate independently, a small

scooter board is utilized to enable him to move around the room. This provides a good means of developing upper extremity use which is vital for future crutch walking. For the child who is just beginning to move around independently on his stomach, a scooter board is a useful device to facilitate locomotion (Finnie, 1970). Slight effort causes movement which might not have been otherwise possible and the child experiences mobility and a sense of competence in his own ability to create the movement. For the child who is just beginning to move around on his stomach, his need for the security of the floor where he can control his own locomotion may temporarily preclude use of the scooter board. However, as his confidence increases, he will welcome the introduction of a scooter board as a means of more rapid locomotion.

To the one-year-old child who is ready for independent walking, the repeated falls when learning to walk hold no fear. To the older child of two or three years of age, walking alone can produce fear. Therapist, teachers and parents must be aware of this and not insist that the child constantly try to take steps unassisted. A child can be encouraged to walk by having an adult hold both hands, then gradually give only one hand support. As the child becomes more secure in this manner of walking, a stick or a doll can be used with the child holding one end and the adult holding the other. It is really a weaning process from holding a hand to holding something less secure and requires the child to advance gradually to supporting himself (Finnie, 1970).

A one-year-old whose maturational development follows a normal pattern often takes his first unsteady steps to the outstretched arms of his mother or father. The parent's delight, coupled with the baby's pleasure with himself, reinforces a desire to repeat the performance whenever his father or mother hold out their arms and call to him. Because walking is usually delayed for the handicapped child, and his body tends to be less predictable and less responsive to his desires, he may be more fearful and his parents' anxiety may be more intense. Under these circumstances, to urge the child to walk from one adult to another presents no particular incentive for the child,

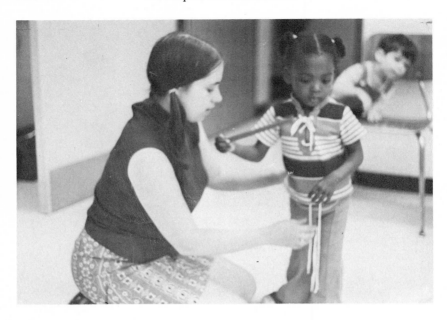

intensifies his fear, and serves to satisfy the adults' needs rather than the child's.

Gross motor activity is scheduled for fifteen minutes of each session. The equipment used, a large red and white ball, a slide, empty boxes, a barrel, and tires on rollers are attractive and exciting to the children so that as soon as they are brought into the room the class expresses delight and responds by walking or crawling to them. The staff responds to the children's anticipation by asking, for example, "Who wants to go on the ball?" The children take turns sitting on the ball, lying on it on their stomachs and on their backs. The ball is a means of giving a child a sense of relation of his body to space. He can be placed on it and rolled so that he lands first on his hands to elicit a protective reaction as he reaches forward, and then he can be rolled back so that he lands on his feet to elicit weight bearing (Seman, 1967). The rocking motion inhibits spasticity, encourages the use of both hands, and exposes the child to a new kind of movement.

Sitting in the tire mounted on casters encourages sitting

balance, or, with the child on his stomach, the tire can be used in the same way as a scooter board as the child learns to propel himself by pushing with his arms. With sides of the tire providing security and support children develop equilibrium response when they are whirled gently across the room.

Crawling through the barrel provides movement through an enclosure. Large empty cartons to curl up in, a sliding board to climb up and slide down all provide a variety of motor experiences and a discovery of the relationship of one's body to space.

ACTIVITIES TO DEVELOP FINE MOTOR SKILLS

In the normally developing fetus the earliest manifestation of gross motor activity is the movement of the limbs in flexion and extension (Gillette, 1969). The infant engages in many random movements such as kicking the legs and opening and closing the hands as though rehearsing for the mastery of more complex motor skills which have yet to appear. The kicking of the legs simultaneously and in reciprocal movement are the forerunners of walking. The random hand movements of infancy are followed by gross motor activities such as grasping and releasing with the use of fingers and palm, often not utilizing the thumb at all. Grasping with fingers and thumb signifies a step toward find coordination because fine motor skill requires control of all the fingers and the wrist in movement and coordination as in accomplishing the specific tasks of picking up small objects between the thumb and index finger. The acquisition of this skill is necessary for self-feeding, buttoning and shoe lacing (McGraw, 1963).

Encouraging use of the hands in all types of activities and with all kinds of materials is important in developing fine motor skills in all children. Handicapped children especially should be participants rather than observers. Because many activities are difficult for the physically involved child, games and toys chosen for him frequently require only that he watch passively. Instead, children should be put on the floor and encouraged to explore objects as to their quality, shape, and

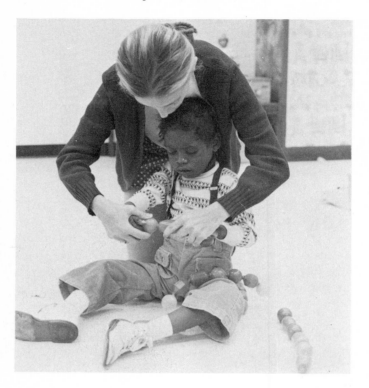

texture. Care must be exercised in the choice of toys because the young child places objects in his mouth as a means of familiarizing himself with them. This is a normal developmental procedure and if toys are chosen carefully, need not be forbidden.

When children have learned to grasp and release, they pick up an object and then drop it. This can be observed with food and eating utensils as well as with toys. The next step is usually to grasp an item, put it into a container and then remove it. Children will be content to repeat this routine for long periods as they engage themselves in the practice of the motor activity of grasp and release and in the acquisition of the concept of a smaller object fitting into a larger one.

Nesting toys of various sizes, large round pegs and a peg board, or a box to serve as a "garage" and a number of small cars and trucks provide the children with long periods of enjoyment and stimulate them to continue a meaningful learning experience.

Balls of various sizes and textures are sometimes put on the floor in the classroom. A large rubber ball, a medium size terry cloth ball and a homemade nylon-filled ball encourage the child to touch and throw even if they are not yet ready to engage in a reciprocal game of "catch" with an adult. Soft cuddly dolls and hard plastic cars and trucks are available to provide tactile stimulation. The occupational therapist brings in a box containing scraps of velvet, terry cloth and sandpaper which are handed out for the child to feel and to rub on his cheek or stomach. The hard cold glass of the windows and the soft warmth of the carpet are always available for exploration. Finger play and paints provide additional manipulating experiences.

RESPONSE AND INITIATION

As the therapist observed the child's locomotion patterns and the manner in which he manipulates his body to achieve mobility, she finds many opportunities to "plug in" to his activities. As Karl crept laboriously to interest centers and to the snack table in the classroom, he pushed on his elbows to achieve locomotion without the use of his legs. To develop strength in the scapular muscles and to facilitate him and knee flexion, the therapist first provided resistance by holding his legs. Then she lifted his pelvis to facilitate hip and knee flexion (amphibian reaction) and applied firm pressure to the soles of his feet thus facilitating extension. Now Karl uses a swimming motion to move across the floor.

Gerald usually crawls in a tripedal fashion, weight bearing on one arm and dragging the spastic arm. The therapist facilitates weight bearing on the involved arm by applying scapular pressure. She does this by bearing down or by bouncing his arm. Then she opens his hand and strokes it to enhance its use. When Jeff initiates ball playing with the teacher, he sits on his heels. As Jeff is engrossed in rolling and catching the ball, the physical therapist places his legs in Indian position, then sits behind him and rocks his knees to stretch the adductor muscles. Rather than imposing arbitrary activities and positioning, the physical therapist takes her cues from the child's current interests and level of functioning.

FACILITATING EMERGING BEHAVIOR

Because mothers observe a child's behavior from day to day, they are known to exclaim, "Today he tried to crawl," or "She's trying to reach her toys." This emerging behavior in the handicapped child should be encouraged by putting the child in the position that will allow him the optimal opportunity to perform. Because of the child's physical limitations, the adults working with him must be especially observant of emerging behaviors so that they can present him with opportunities to facilitate accomplishment.

When treating a handicapped child, the staff is always aware of the level at which the child is functioning. This pertains to his physical, social, cognitive and emotional development. A child may be functioning at his chronological age mentally but not physically. For example, he may have limited use of his legs but be proficient in language skills.

As the therapist charts the initial evaluation, she notes those activities that the child accomplished independently, those with which the child needs some assistance, those that are just emerging and those that he cannot do at all. The therapist begins therapy at the functioning level at which she first sees the child. It should be noted that the word activities is used rather than skills because an activity may be a skill or a part of a skill.

To facilitate an emerging behavior, a child must be encouraged to perform in such a manner as to take him on toward the next skill or activity. If a child has mastered the skill of sitting on the floor using his hands for support, then the next procedure would be to get the child to balance himself with one hand support so that he can use the other hand to reach for a toy. In line with this thought, a child will sit unsupported for a few seconds when he is engrossed in watching the therapist or another child. A therapist will use this technique at the beginning while the child is unaware of his achievement. It is understood that the skill is not fully internalized until the child is able to sit unsupported at will.

A physically handicapped child learns skills at a slower rate than the normal child. He may learn to sit but the time required for him to master the skill is longer than it is for the average child. Yet it is important that the handicapped child be assisted to the sitting position and supported if necessary if he is expected to attempt to do so on his own initiative.

A child can be placed in a sitting position with too much support. The child who is able to support his own head should be allowed to hold his own head erect. For the child with head and shoulder control, a tie across the waist or between the legs is sufficient. For short periods of time the therapist will concentrate on sitting activity without the tie. She may suggest to the teachers and parents that some time should be allowed the child to sit without the tie as long as someone is nearby to prevent falls. This can be gratifying experience for the child. When Beth is seated at the table for snack, the tie is brought up between her legs to stabilize her hips, but she is not tied so completely that she does not have the use of her own body to keep her balance.

Children who are chronologically beyond the age of learning to sit but who have not yet mastered this skill often spend too much time lying on their backs. When the therapist places them on their stomachs or in a sitting position, they sometimes voice their objections by crying or by throwing themselves backwards. Children may fear a new position because they cannot alter the position or because the world has a different and unfamiliar look from the new position. It may take time and patience for the child to become accustomed to the new position. The child who dislikes sitting at first may learn to sit independently and enjoy it. The child who resents being on his stomach at first may soon adjust and begin to pull himself along the floor.

As the handicapped child develops, he needs many experiences within his capabilities and a few that are slightly beyond his capabilities. Because his disability causes him to be more dependent on adults than the average child, therapist, teacher and parents must remain alert to emerging behavior.

Therapy is meant to help a child to reach his maximum potential according to his physical, mental and emotional capabilities. In regard to a child's physical disability, one must be aware of the severity of the disability and not have unrealistic expectations. Ambulating independently may not be the goal for every child, but rather self-care, be it from an upright position or from a wheelchair. The most important therapy goal for the handicapped child is that he be able to care for his own needs in order to achieve the greatest measure of independence possible for him, for it is through mastery of activities of daily living that he will begin to view himself as someone of value.

CHAPTER 9

PROMOTING SELF-AWARENESS
AND BODY MASTERY

AWARENESS OF SELF is the *sine qua non* of humanness. As a
young child explores, gaining feedback from his environment, each message he receives about objects and their
properties carries with it a message about the child himself. In
early childhood, and indeed throughout life, physical and later
language transactions between child and environment are processed in terms both of objective knowledge and subjective
experience.

It is characteristic of early sensorimotor schemata, according
to Piaget, that the child is able to separate neither himself nor
his own action from the physical object upon which the action is
performed. Representational thought, to which the child normally accedes during about the third year of life, is marked by
the acquisition of symbolic functioning, that is, by the child's
newly gained knowledge of the distinction between symbol and
referent. Through this ability, he is able to represent, or construct within his mind, external events. This inner psychic
reality, thought, ultimately reaches its apex during adolescence
with the beginning of formal operations, which enable the
individual to consider and to analyze his own reasoning process. As is the case during earlier stages of development, that
new ability, too, is accompanied by a form of egocentrism, a
subjectivism, with pronounced affective concomitants, but
rooted in the individual's mode of thought.

Much has been written about the contributions of experiences during the preschool years toward the formation of
self-concept. During the third and fourth years, the child becomes increasingly aware of himself as a distinct entity, with
characteristics, powers and limitations, such as the limitation of
size as he compares himself with important others. Through
the process of comparison of himself with others in his ex-

periential world, he gains at least a rudimentary understanding of concepts such as those involving the dichotomies of living vs. non-living things, male vs. female, and large vs. small. In a sense, the child becomes increasingly his own frame of reference for internalizing knowledge gained through each new experience. The more he learns about objects, persons, and phenomena processed through his active mental experience, the more he learns, and becomes able to imagine, about himself.

Normal concerns about body integrity experienced by young children have been effectively described by Selma Fraiberg (1959). The propensity for magical thinking, interacting with newly acquired awareness of self, may serve to generate powerful fantasies concerning imminent loss of a body part, for example. Emma Plank (1962, 1963) has described the need to attend to the fantasies and fears of a hospitalized child and the educational and supportive role of the Child Life Educator in a hospital setting.

Subjective experiences, such as those of comfort and safety, of anxiety and dread, are important motivational determinants for early learning. Of particular importance is the feedback to the child concerning his own sense of efficacy. Beyond the realm of affect itself, relating to the child's gratification concerning his own competence, power and accomplishment, and to his feelings of self-worth and adequacy, is the important cognitive component of awareness of causality. Learning that things have causes and consequences during this period of development is spurred on by the child's wishes to feel competent and to test the limits of his own power to produce effect upon his physicosocial environment. Thus, thought and feeling, physical knowledge and self-attitudes, are reciprocal. A child learns about causal relations through activity in which he is centrally involved.

Young handicapped children are often observed at a particular disadvantage in these action-dependent learning modes. The child with spina bifida, for example, with the advent of the shunting procedure, no longer is necessarily doomed to probable hydrocephalitic retardation and short life expectancy, and he may even develop rather precociously intellectual compensations for his physical limitations. It is not unusual for these children to become unduly passive with respect to physical activity, if manipulating adults around them have a highly unpleasant and demanding manner. Jill, whose language development was suspected to be potentially adequate for her age, was at first most negativistic and resistant to adults' attempts to get her to perform a task. These exchanges were usually punctuated by loud whining and occasionally by screaming. Initially, Jill seemed totally uninterested in classroom toys, often to the point of complete lethargy. In time she would attempt a task, but only when held by an adult. Her language behavior, usually inappropriate and echolalic, came increasingly to resemble a game she played with adults. This is suggested in the following anecdote from the teacher's daily record summary.

> In July, she played a verbal game with an adult in which she contradicted the adult's *yes* or *no* with her own. Three times she was able to respond *yes, yes, yes* to the adult's *no, no, no*. She laughed and thoroughly enjoyed the game.

The first step toward the development of both purposive thought and self-concept is the differentiation of self from other. According to Piaget, early in life the child fails to distinguish between his action and the object upon which he acts. Acquisition of the object concept enables him to apprehend objects as entities, the existence of which is independent of his own action. Thus, the self comes to be distinguished from the rest of the environment as objects in the environment are distinguished as *permanent,* discrete entities.

Affectively, H. S. Sullivan (1953) noted that social interactions both facilitate such differentiation and color it with a feeling tone. Thus, *good breast—bad breast* as an important dimension of experience brings about a self-evaluative dimension of subjective experience: *good me—bad me.* The process of *separation—individuation,* with its libidinal and cognitive components, has been formulated as a theory from the psychoanalytic perspective by Margaret Mahler (1965).

Acquisition of an initial concept of self, the most basic concept and reference point, perhaps, for all subsequent learning, is accomplished through the coordination of sensorimotor schemas. Afferent and efferent processes, in interaction and through successively more complex organization, provide the child with the information he needs in order to locate himself in space, establish body boundaries, and ultimately to act on the basis of intention and purpose.

Sensory information is taken in through visual, auditory, tactile, and other channels and provides the basis for action, during the first year or so, for increasingly more complex and adaptive applications of reflex patterns. One important source of data needed for the establishment of the location of the body in space is provided by the vestibular mechanism. Work with young cerebral palsied children must often first begin with activities which enable the child to achieve positional balance, to experience sensations of rolling, sitting upright, or walking on knees, not only for the purpose of strengthening and relaxing muscles, but perhaps more basically to activate antigravity muscle systems and to provide sensation concerning altered body orientation in space, positional stability, and movement. Through such activities the child can experience his own body and can learn to activate and inhibit body movement in response to gravity.

Under the guidance of the physical therapist, HEED staff incorporates a variety of activities in the classroom setting which are intended to assist children in gaining body orientation and sensation of altered position and movement. Many of these were discussed more fully in Chapter 8, with the note that most such activities are actually multipurpose. They enable children to interact with each other and with one or more adults; hence, they are social in nature, often requiring the child to exercise a degree of trust in others. Many are intended to relax specific muscle systems or to strengthen certain large muscles. Cause and effect understandings may also come about at such times, often as incidental learning gained in a play context. Perhaps more importantly, however, being rolled on a sheet or stretched across the large ball, crawling through a tunnel, and climbing up the stairs and descending the slide are activities which provide new body sensations, perceptible changes in body orientation in space, the experience of movement, and the like. Such sensations contribute greatly to the establishment of body image and body schema.

DEVELOPING COMPETENCE IN ACTIVITIES
OF DAILY LIVING

The concept of activities of daily living, or ADL, suggests the major role of the occupational therapist in work with young handicapped children. Feeding, toileting, dressing and undressing are areas of intense concern to parents and to the child himself, whose view of self and feelings of mastery are to a high degree dependent upon the success he experiences in these areas. It is frequently difficult to determine precisely where the concerns of the occupational therapist and those of the physical therapist, speech pathologist, and teacher can be distinguished, if indeed they are distinguishable at all. In her glossary of *Terminology for Parents,* Finnie (1968) defines occupational therapy as "treatment given to improve movement for daily living."

In Project HEED, the occupational therapist serves the vital role of relating to parents around techniques which they might use at home in handling such areas as eating and elimination. Such guidance is based upon both the therapist's own diagnostic evaluation and on-going study of and experience with the child and the detailed observations supplied by the teacher, physical therapist, and teaching assistant. Often, techniques such as gradually increasing the density of soft foods, such as oatmeal, through mixing in more solid food items were first tried in the classroom and then recommended for home application. Parents' needs in such areas as this simply cannot be overstated, and most HEED parents conveyed an awareness that their own tension and anxiety concerning them was readily conveyed to the child. With respect to self-care and maintenance of body functions with minimal stress, success is always shared by all three: the child, his parents, and the staff.

FEEDING: A SPECIAL AREA

Snack time has traditionally occupied an important place in nursery education. In most cultures eating is at least in part a social activity, a time for sharing. The circle format characterizing family mealtime permits face to face contact, and consequently, at least visual communication if not always verbal sharing.

The delegation of responsibilities by individuals for the welfare of the group surrounding snack time, or now in many programs for young children lunch or breakfast, is assumed to create an awareness of one's identity as a member of a social group, the nursery school class. The obvious sense of pride in accomplishment experienced by many if not most preschoolers who help to serve, to set the table, to pour juice, or to pass the wastebasket for clean up at snack time suggests the salience of this activity for the child's development of self-esteem.

For many physically handicapped children, feeding has been an especially difficult, often painful, area. Frequently, handicapped children show little interest in eating. Through cooperative effort of teacher, parent, occupational therapist and speech pathologist, several HEED children had to be taught to swallow. The lack of normal feedback from stimulation of the tongue, for example, might lead the child to pro-trude his tongue when fed. Considering the stressful times experienced by many parents of non-handicapped toddlers surrounding feeding, it is not surprising that both the handicapped child and his parents often find mealtime the most difficult of all. Therefore, help for the child (and his parents) with food intake is intrinsically a priority item for many children.

Behind this, however, Erik Erikson has related the social modality of taking in (i.e. love, visual and tactile sensations, information) to Freud's view of the oral stage as the first of several psychosexual stages. The mouth and its related internal and external tissues comprise an erogenous zone, a locus of concentration of libido. Through his experiences during the first major period of life, the infant establishes a mode of responding to the world along the dimension of Basic Trust vs. Basic Mistrust. This aspect of *ego identity,* as Erikson terms it, is one of several encountered sequentially throughout the life cycle. Identity, or personality more generally, is not fully formed as a result of the experiences the child must integrate during the oral, anal, and phallic stages, climaxed by the oedipal conflict and resolution, according to Erikson. However, the prime time for resolution of each of the eight crises Erikson identifies is in general age-related, and the crises are sequential.

Many HEED children, entering the program during the second year of life, would have had difficulty dealing with the developmental tasks Erikson associates with the oral period. Rather than having progressed to a more active, aggressive mode of oral activity (getting and holding), which normally accompanies dentition, many of these children exercise little if any voluntary control over food intake. Whether such limitations, and the concomitant social responses of mothers and fathers to them, may have far-reaching deleterious effects on the development of a sense of self, a positive yet realistically adaptive world view, and diverse aspects of personality formation, is assumed to remain in the theoretical sphere.

ASSERTION OF OWNERSHIP AND INTENTION

Both possessive assertions and indications of intent or purpose are hallmarks of autonomy. Bettelheim (1967) has noted among older autistic children the absence of assertion of ownership, both behaviorally and linguistically. Intention, identified by Piaget as the beginning of intelligence, is related also to the subjective experience of autonomy and effectiveness. Each of these areas was identified as a primary target for intervention in the HEED program.

Perhaps the most important single feature of a peer group learning experience for two and three-year-old physically handicapped children is the opportunity it creates and constantly maintains for growth in the ability to assert one's own will and rights in the face of threat from one or more peers.

Tammy, for example, although aware of peers, was at first able to maintain a high degree of psychological isolation from them except at snack time. After several experiences of having a cookie snatched, the teacher saying, "Tell him 'No! Don't take my cookie!' " Tammy began to pull her cookie out of an encroaching child's reach, sometimes forming the word or even softly uttering, "No." The teacher's task is to use such incidents positively, in terms of guiding both aggressor and victim, so that both gain an understanding of the rights and requisites of ownership.

This scenario is played out almost daily at snack time, an ideal situation for channeling such incidents in positive directions since the teacher can become directly involved from the beginning of the incident. No effort is made, therefore, to prevent such happenings by, for example, maintaining greater distance between children, separating the aggressive from the meek or otherwise seeking to avoid situations which, if exploited, can be excellent learning and growth opportunities.

Such opportunities present themselves, also, in the context of manipulative play with materials in the room. The passive child who begins to engage in desultory manipulation of a toy car, a plastic hammer or other play item, only to relinquish it without protest to a peer, must be helped through patient guidance and with small steps to come at last to the ability to protect and keep what is his. With very young handicapped children, words alone are insufficient; actions must accompany them as staff members attempt to encourage assertiveness. Instant judgments are constantly required as to whether the snatched item should be reclaimed for the child, or whether such external intervention may serve to reinforce passivity and dependence.

Just as intentionality observed in a child's play signals the emergence of intelligence, so it suggests the establishment of autonomy and will. A child may not be able to say, "I'm going to play with the sand," but he may in many other ways reveal the formation of an intent, the selection of a means, and the determination to achieve a goal.

A number of activities and media serve to foster the child's awareness of self. A favorite singing game, for example, is

"Jack in the Box." In this game, usually played in the moments before snack is served, the children are seated around a semicircular table, facing the teacher, who leads the singing and acting out of the game:

> Jack in the box
> Sits so still
> Won't you come out?
> *Yes,* I will!

Teacher and children lower heads and cover eyes, only to pop up on the last line. The game is played over and over, and several parents have reported it is spontaneously played at home. The "Jack in the Box" game probably draws its appeal from several sources. First, it is akin to the "peek" game of infancy. A young child, beginning to acquire the concept of the permanent object, is delighted to find his parent still there when he uncovers his eyes. His egocentrism is apparent in the impression one gets that he believes himself invisible when he, ostrich style, covers his eyes. There is, in any case, an element of surprise giving way to expectation. The game persists as long as there continues to be any uncertainty concerning its outcome.

The appeal of ritual-like singing games to young children is well known, especially if augmented by physical movement in the form of interpretive action. Probably both the predictability of the routine and the build-up to a climax, which continues to appear novel even after countless repetitions, contribute to the pleasure HEED children have found in the "Jack in the Box" game. Probably, too, both the shared nature of the activity and the focus of attention upon the experience of seeing and being seen, not to mention the experience of acting out a role in a form of dramatic play, have implication for the growth of a sense of self.

BODY AWARENESS AND IDENTIFICATION

The ability to derive feedback from physical movement and from contact with the environment is generally to some degree impaired in the handicapped child. Unable to feel the floor beneath his feet, he may resist standing with assistance or independently. Other tactile sensation deficits or impairments interfere, directly or indirectly, with speech and with food intake, and uncontrolled drooling may be present. Goals in increasing sensory input, after first determining the child's threshold of sensory experience especially through the tactile modality, are established. Commonly accepted special therapy techniques of brushing, manipulating, and applying ice to the mouth area are used in order to alter sensory thresholds in preparation for eating, speech facilitation, and other activities.

Working with media such as finger paints or similar materials provides opportunities for increasing tactile experience, thus enhancing both the ability and the willingness to experience tactile sensations, as well as gradually to learn to discriminate among sensations. Thus, although a rudimentary sense of pride in accomplishment with the product may be possible as very young handicapped children work at creative projects, growth in sense of self often must also occur at a much more basic level of sensory and kinesthetic functioning.

An index of a child's progress in achieving an accurate and complete concept of self is his manifest knowledge of body

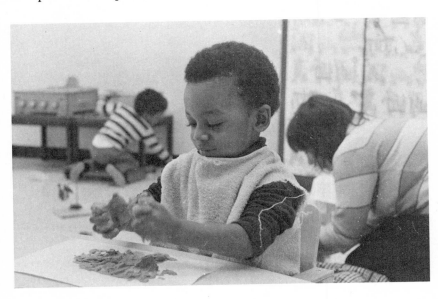

parts. A great many traditional parent–infant games ("Where's your nose?") are directed toward this end. In the HEED program, the teacher attempted to inventory periodically the child's ability to identify correctly body parts, and each child's progress was carefully recorded.

With somewhat older children, self-drawings can serve to indicate the maturity (i.e. completeness and accuracy) and even the affective quality of a child's concept of self. (See, for example, DiLeo, 1970; Kellogg, 1967; Lowenfeld and Brittain, 1964.) Prior to this evidence of mental representation of self, however, recognition of self can be demonstrated, even without the aid of speech.

In addition to the child's recognition of discrete components, recognition of self as a gestalt is an important area of work with all young children, but especially with the handicapped or otherwise developmentally impaired. The ability of the child to recognize his own mirror reflection, a photograph of himself, and his own image and actions presented via a videotape monitor is considered basic to the affective evaluation he comes to place upon himself. A child's photograph displayed on the wall, along with his fingerpainting or other creative project, together with consistently addressing him by name, can convey to a child not only who he is but that he is *somebody.*

An item of basic importance in terms of the acquisition of self-awareness is a mirror. On many occasions, the teacher, occupational therapist, or other staff member may wish to use a small hand mirror in working with the child in areas such as those related to eating and talking. The child's attention may thus be focused directly on a part of his body, and he can come to observe his own mastication. The small mirror has the advantage of permitting focus on a discrete area and activity and is useful if the facial area is to be targeted.

Otherwise, a full-length wall mirror provides an opportunity for the child to view his entire body, to observe effects of body movements, and the like. Sometimes a child, who is able to sit unattended or who can be placed in a bolster, may explore visually before a mirror for some time. Other children, a teacher, therapist, or a parent in the classroom may support a

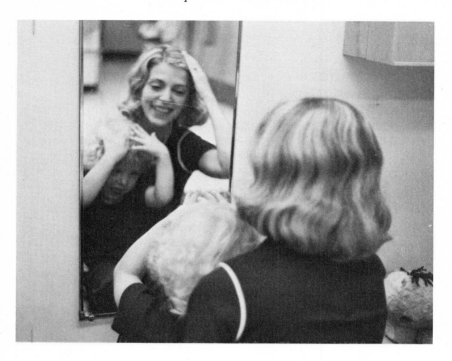

child and talk to him about the image before them. It is often useful for a child to observe himself in the act of pointing to named body parts or to play a hand-clapping game with the adult. Adults often fail to realize that for a young child, particularly if he is handicapped, seeing himself in a mirror may be a very novel experience. The small child will not, of course, immediately realize that it is he himself who is reflected in the mirror. But with this realization comes a host of new discoveries, and perhaps the very beginning awareness that he has objective form and exists as an entity among numerous other entities in the environment.

Adults, of course, must attempt to gauge the extent of the child's discoveries, the level of curiosity, and the quality of awareness in order to use such learning opportunities most effectively. There is a time for adult verbalization and a time for uninterrupted discovery.

REPRESENTATIONAL PLAY AND SENSE OF SELF

Just as with all children, housekeeping play or other dramatic modes provide opportunities not only for cognitive growth but for a particular aspect of such growth: development of a concept of self. Such play is, therefore, imitative, often incorporating the child's interpretive translations of what he sees mother do. Other adults, including fathers, soon come to be imitated too, and diverse roles may be played out in such play. Normally, dramatic play conveying mothering, family, and work themes begins to appear consistently among threes and fours, although precursors are apparent in earlier spontaneous play. One important precursor, deferred imitation, indicates the child's readiness to engage in true symbolic thought.

Not all children are equally able to initiate and to participate in dramatic play as Smilansky (1968) has shown. In her work with disadvantaged non-European Israeli children, Smilansky found that such play behavior had to be taught, and, indeed, that it could be taught. As was suggested earlier in this book, the concept experientially deprived can provide a rubric for a variety of handicapping conditions, those relating to deficiencies in the environmental opportunities available to a child as well as those due to a child's inability to interact fully or optimally with his environment.

It is the interaction between mental structure and environmental condition or experience which enables a child to evolve more complex structure and, consequently, to manifest more versatile and sophisticated skills. This suggests that simply to provide experiences and assume that development will proceed perforce is insufficient. Each experience must be geared to the child's present level of functioning. Consequently, the appearance of deferred imitation may signal that a child is able to represent internally an object or experience.

An activity which has appeared to elicit a degree of representational play in a number of children involves the use of a large, plastic, boat-shaped tub. Young children's water play is always an interesting activity to observe, and may provide many avenues for cognitive growth. The fascination, and sometimes the anxiety, water elicits in young children is commonly noted. The teacher remembered the tub during a session in which two or three children were being encouraged to play with dolls, with verbalized descriptions of the dolls as "babies." The tub was brought in and, with approximately five inches of water in it, allowed the children to reach the water while seated or kneeling beside the tub. Beth was able to use the water by lying supine on a bench of the same height as the tub.

Apparently, this activity serves to encourage dramatic play enactments of "giving baby a bath." Soap was introduced, and each child became engrossed in scrubbing, sudsing, and rinsing, then towel-drying a doll. The activity soon attracted other children, of both sexes, and each had an area in which to work and a doll to bathe. Play patterns were definitely parallel, and the activity appeared to mean very different things to different children. However, a degree of identification with the doll seemed to characterize the play of nearly every child, together with some apparent instances of deferred imitation expressed through solicitous mothering behavior.

Water play, whether of this nature or developed in other directions by the children themselves, appears never to lose its novelty. It is a medium which seems to elicit representational behavior as well as sensory exploration. Through bathing a doll, a child may take the role of parent, assign the doll the role of a child, and consequently, be able to see elements of both self and parent more sharply and to express these through play. Even body form itself may come into a clearer focus when one is administering a bath.

In Project HEED, the special expertise of each discipline is brought to bear and orchestrated in order to foster the total development of each child within the limits imposed by his handicap. And a central and unifying theme in this effort is concern that the child will grow in awareness and positive evaluation of himself as a competent and valued individual who can come to terms both with himself and his handicap and with the physicosocial world of his experience.

Whereas this chapter and the one which preceded it reflect the necessary focus on the individual child and the individualization of staff efforts required to foster his physical and personal growth, the chapter which follows addresses the social milieu in which such individualization occurs. A value traditionally ascribed to early education programs is their role in fostering the socialization of the young child, in providing a means by which he can learn to accommodate his own needs to those of others and to gain skills in social interaction within a peer setting. That such social development and individual personal growth are reciprocal is a theme of the discussion which follows and represents the rationale for the group program which was implemented in this project.

CHAPTER 10

PROMOTING PEER AWARENESS AND SOCIAL INTERACTION

THE SOCIALIZING AIMS of early education programs have traditionally been given recognition and priority. A nursery school child of three or four may begin his school experiences fearfully, separating from his mother with considerable difficulty, and, although manifesting varying degrees of interest in his peers, will generally require some time to accommodate to these new surroundings. There is considerable question concerning the ability of the three or even four-year-old to engage in truly cooperative play, to know and to appreciate what sharing means, and to grasp the understanding that others, peers and the adult teacher, have needs and wishes of their own. The egocentrism of this age may bind the child too firmly to permit the development of true social reciprocity. This issue may hinge mainly on one's definition of concepts such as empathy and egocentrism, however, and to what extent, if at all, they are mutually exclusive.

A social sense of some form is observed emerging in the course of young children's nursery experience by most, if not all, of their teachers. The nursery school experiences, social and cognitive, may well be, in many, many instances, reinforcing trends and learnings well established in the child's home environment and in the neighborhood. It is usually not believed that a child is placed in a social milieu only during the hours of his nursery school attendance, spending the remainder of his time in psychological isolation.

Those areas in which participation in an early education experience are assumed to foster the development of a young child as a social being include such diverse purposes as guidance in the socialization of aggression; gaining some degree of internal regulation of impulses; acquiring efficacy in communication functions; gaining greater cognitive clarity through meaningful learning of self-other similarities and differences; learning about and gaining acceptance of human diversity, among individuals and possibly among racial or other ethnic groups.

The "socialization" aspect of early education includes also the child's learning to use an adult as a resource, to whom he must attend and whom he must share willingly with several others. Typically, the nursery teacher's instructional program balances self-selected activity opportunities, during which children may establish communication links with each other and evolve increasingly social play patterns, with relatively more structured group activities led by the teacher. These latter include group activities such as finger plays, songs, rhythm instruments, eurythmics, story time, and a variety of others, each with its specific purpose and rationale, but all having in common the imposition of social constraints on children. At these times, the children must comprise a group, must attend to the leader (who may be a peer, as well as an adult), must coordinate their individual participation with others.

The group social experiences, however, take many other forms. A child must often be helped to understand that his use of a particular toy must be deferred until a peer is no longer using it, for example. He may become aware that a child is absent, learn that the child is ill, and note when the child returns to nursery school. Occasionally, a classmate may have a misfortune, or become angry or sad. Or a new child may join the class. Usually, consistent play pairings will develop and then become modified. Often friendships will emerge.

Nursery teachers at the Heman Rehabilitation Institute frequently note the dramatic changes observed during the course of a year, not only in the development of individual children, but in the development of a group as a whole. Prior to the initiation of Project HEED, for most of the three and four-year-old children with a variety of physical handicaps, participation in the agency's nursery school program represented the very first exposure to a peer group setting. The child may have been seen at the agency by a physical therapist, but the visit was on an individual basis—much as the child may already have experienced in doctor's examining rooms and hospital clinics. Despite the necessity of such examinations and therapy sessions, and the fact that they may have been of great help to the child, they have provided little pleasure or joy and possibly much pain and stress.

When a newly formed nursery group starts out at the beginning of the year, consisting mainly of former outpatients in physical therapy and other children new to the agency altogether, they comprise a "group" only nominally. Effecting comfortable separation requires, for many children and mothers, patience and careful guidance. Some parents do not understand or are unable to deal with their child's anxieties concerning separation. Many of the children in such a group are incontinent; consequently, the first weeks seem oriented primarily to the development of bathroom and changing routines.

Play behavior may be primitive or seemingly nonexistent, and individual manipulative play with sand, blocks, or puzzles is difficult enough to establish, let alone associative play. Group activities, such as story, music, or snack time, are often chaotic and overwhelming for children and staff alike.

As the year progresses, although achievements of individual children are noted, changes in the social context within which these achievements occur may be overlooked. However, within a few months the group bears little resemblance to the collection of frightened or docile, nonambulatory, soiling and psychologically isolated youngsters observed in September. A sense of community appears to exist. When a new child enters the class, he will be received with much interest. Many children have become almost gregarious and will approach visitors with greetings and questions. The circular snack table signals sharing and mutuality, and children rotate in the role of "snack teacher."

That the same degree of social behavior is attainable earlier in life, especially for children whose primary handicap may be accompanied by pronounced slowness in the development of the social tools of language, is doubtful indeed. The HEED project was not conceived as a readiness program for nursery school. Rather, the rationale for an integrated group program for eighteen through thirty-six month old handicapped children stressed a recognition of the important areas of development associated with this age period. The social behavior of two-year-olds was believed to be qualitatively as well as quantitatively different from that of older children.

For this group, the peer setting was thought to represent a means much more than an end in itself. It was not assumed that HEED children would learn to subordinate their own needs or desires to the well-being of a fellow or of the group as a whole. Rather, the presence of age-mates would create occasion for a child to assert his will, constrained only by those limitations necessary to guarantee the physical and psychological safety of others.

The presence of peers, as with older children, creates opportunities for model emulation. However, for these children, the consistent use of imitation itself as a learning mode was the target, rather than the adoption of desirable behaviors observed in a peer.

At all ages, a social setting provides opportunity for communicative language. In many HEED children the social use of speech theorized by Vigotsky to provide an initial basis for later inner, mediative language functioning, had not developed at all or was present only in primitive and immature form. Speech stimulation was intended to be an important aspect of the HEED classroom, provided not only directly by the adults present, but also by the need to communicate inherent in any human social context, even among two-year-olds.

Self-awareness and body concept development were also believed to be enhanced by the presence of others. If these reflect a child's developing schema of self, the presence of other children may provide opportunities for clarifying and modifying the schema.

COMPOSITION OF THE GROUPS

When Project HEED was initiated, with sixteen children referred by physicians, a decision about grouping was necessary.

Two classes were planned, one to meet on Monday and Wednesday, the other on Tuesday and Thursday, each for a period of two hours. The staff debated the relative merits of two alternative plans. A vertical grouping would allow a greater range in functional level and age differential and the mothers would perhaps benefit from seeing such a range. The mothers of older children would encourage the mothers of younger ones and could themselves become more aware of gains their own child had made.

The other sentiment, and the one finally adopted, was that because the differences in functional levels were so obvious and so pronounced, it would be best to separate the groups by chronological and functional age. It was felt that such a situation would provide more opportunities for peer interaction as well as greater flexibility in daily planning.

Within the first few months developmental and functional differences between the two groups became more apparent and when new children were added, initial gross evaluations were used to place the child accordingly. The staff at this point felt sure that their decision on group placement was the correct one. Those in the Monday-Wednesday group, identified here as Group A, quickly benefited from peer imitation and modeling. Those in Group B benefited from the more intensive help which the staff was able to provide because the needs of each child were so similar.

In the course of the first year the staff became convinced that the children in Group B required a more structured program with objectives quite different from the socializing and peer modeling goals of Group A. At the beginning of the second year of the Project's operation, the children in Group B were involved in a program from which group activities had been eliminated but which provided instead a constant one-to-one relationship with an adult. Teacher, therapist, teacher assistant, and parents each worked with one child throughout the session, providing sensory input, facilitation and relaxation techniques and other appropriate stimuli. The room was bare of all but basic equipment for all but the last twenty minutes of the session, and even then each child was provided with one toy at a time. By restricting options and eliminating extraneous materials, the staff hoped to limit distractibility and to encourage meaningful activity.

Snack time, rather than serving as a social experience, became a time for teaching the children to tolerate foods new to them, to learn to chew, and to drink from a cup. In contrast to Group A, each child in Group B faced an adult instead of joining his peers around the table for snack time.

SEPARATION FROM MOTHERS

With mothers, teacher and therapist present in the room, each child had the option of interacting solely with his mother or engaging in play with a staff member or another child. The children seemed totally oblivious of each other but usually chose a combination of mother and staff member. They would watch a teacher demonstrate a toy, such as the formboard, and then turn to their mothers to share it with them.

Although at first most of the children needed to remain close to their mothers throughout the entire session, after the first month they were all willing to separate from their mothers at least for brief periods. At first mothers were encouraged to leave the room just long enough to go to the kitchen for a cup of coffee. At the teacher's suggestion, before leaving they always told their children, "I am going to get a cup of coffee and I'll be right back." To inform their children of their intention of leaving and returning seemed to be a new experience for some of the parents and often the statement was made self-consciously and awkwardly. With the teacher available to comfort the child who needed reassurance and to remind him of his mother's promise that she would return, all of the children were soon able to separate from their mothers for increasingly longer periods of time.

When the caseworker began conducting group sessions, only occasionally did a mother have to leave the parent meeting to return to her child. The mother's verbal communication of her intent to leave and her promise to return coupled with the reiteration and reassurance of another adult enabled the children to cope with their separation anxieties.

USES OF SNACK TIME

Although the sessions were still relatively unstructured and the staff took their cues from the children, snack time was scheduled for 10:15 each morning. The children came to the table where they were served cookies and milk. Significantly, peer interactions in Group A were first initiated at snack time. There were instances of one child inadvertently taking another child's cookie and being greeted with a scream of protest. Before long, several children became adept at removing cookies in a teasing manner in order to provoke a protest. They would wait patiently until the child sitting next to them was distracted and then would quickly remove his cookie and hold it aloft. No child in this group was so passive that he permitted this without trying to regain what was rightfully his by grabbing for it, or by protesting to the teacher or both.

The teacher mediated these altercations. "This cookie is yours; this one is Johnny's cookie." However, she was aware of the fact that there was a positive quality to this interaction which snack time evoked and she quickly utilized it to introduce group participation activities. When all the children were seated at the table and before the snack was served, she began teaching simple rhythms: "Touch, touch, touch the table, touch the table together." Some children immediately imitated her hand movements, others merely observed her and many of the children watched their peers. As they all became involved in the game, they pounded the table exuberantly. In subsequent sessions the teacher added body parts: "Touch, touch, touch your head," then "nose," "eyes," and "ears." And "Clap, clap, clap your hands," which proved to be a great favorite.

The next step was to flick the lights on and off to announce snack time. Immediately eight little ones disengaged themselves from other activities to move toward the table. And then clean-up time was added. The lights flicked on and off, the

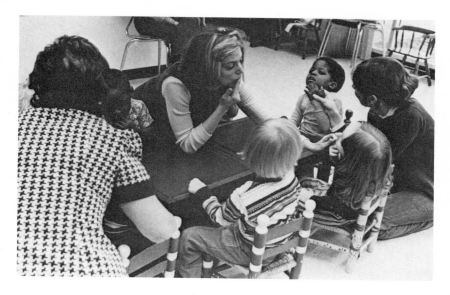

staff sang, "It's clean-up time, it's clean-up time. Time to put the toys away," and immediately the staff began picking up toys from the floor, removing them from the tables and placing them on the cupboard shelves. A few children responded by imitating, the others were encouraged to help in the group effort. Immediately after the toys were removed, everyone chose a chair and pushed it to the table. The physical therapist taught each child how to get himself from the floor to the chair unassisted or with minimal assistance.

As the parents observed this part of the program, they expressed surprise at the rapidity with which the children assimilated the directions, the "rules," and at their capacity to learn self-help skills and to join in group activities.

The children in Group B were more limited motorically and required more adult assistance in all phases of the program. Snack time was signalled by flicking the lights on and off, but few children in this group were able to hold a toy, crawl to the cupboard, and replace the item on the shelf. The teacher encouraged children to lift the toy from the floor and hand it to her. The physical therapist helped those children who were ready to move short distances toward the table.

Many of the children in this group needed help in learning to hold the cookie, to chew and to swallow solid foods, and to drink from a cup. Mothers had been bringing bottles of milk to class and the staff secured their cooperation in not feeding their children during the class session. At snack time, therefore, all the children were thirsty and were eager for the milk. The cup, containing a small amount of liquid, was held by an adult and the child was encouraged to hold the cup and to drink from it. The messiness caused by milk spilling on the table or dribbling down chins was ignored, but whenever a child successfully swallowed some portion of the liquid, he was praised for his accomplishment and many of the children first learned to drink from a cup at snack time.

The parents, who observed with keen interest the staff's efforts at teaching self-feeding, often gave helpful suggestions and a give and take developed between parents and staff. Snack time brought the beginnings of self-feeding skills and mothers were encouraged to try placing small bits of meat, vegetables and fruit in front of the children at mealtimes. Small successes at home were reported and shared by the parents.

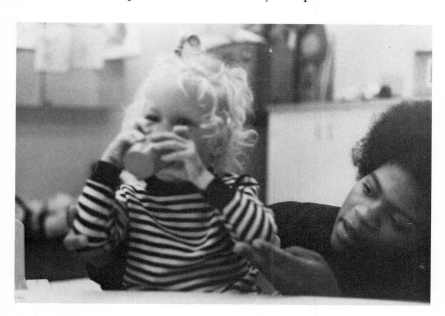

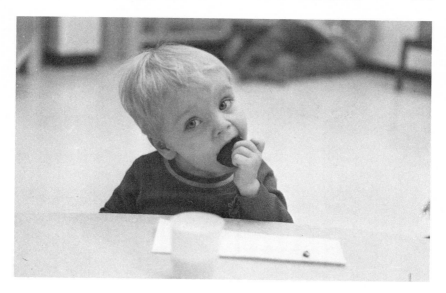

For the children in Group B, snack time was not yet a time for socialization and peer interaction; it was utilized for the learning of basic self-feeding skills.

AWARENESS OF OTHERS

The teacher took an unposed full view snapshot of each child shortly after the child entered the program. The child's photograph and mirror reflection were used initially to detect and subsequently to foster self-awareness. All of the children soon recognized not only their own pictures but spontaneously identified the photographs of classmates. Taking her cues from the children, the teacher began presenting the photos to the children, often as a group activity, and inquiring: "Whose picture is this?" or the open-ended "This is a picture of . . . ." Those who were verbal called out the names and the rest pointed to the appropriate child.

This level of peer awareness was surprising because at first even Johnny, the most intellectually capable child and the one who had experienced no separation anxieties and who had readily accepted the teacher, had been totally oblivious of peers. Three months after the program began he not only knew the names of all his classmates, but could correctly identify each mother-child dyad. On David's first day at the Agency Nursery School, before he actually entered the classroom, David spontaneously identified from photographs mounted above their lockers four former HEED classmates.

Sometimes, as a teacher encouraged a child who was showing interest in building blocks a second child would join them and add to the block structure. When the teacher withdrew, the second child would remain and the two would continue with the block play. Although there was usually no verbal exchange and no seeming awareness of each other, both children would continue to attend to the task.

One day Tommy was lying on his side running a small car back and forth on the floor. David crawled to within inches of him, picked up another car and proceeded to move it up and down in the same pattern. Neither child gave any evidence of awareness of the other as they quietly engaged in solitary play. Slowly David's car went far enough to touch Tommy's and then moved back. This sequence was repeated several times.

After the first month of the program, it was not unusual for one child to seize another child's toy. A yelp of protest often sent the intruder scooting away, but sometimes the interloper took over the play activity, actually shouldering the first child out of the immediate area. At first some of the children accepted these aggressive acts with little or no protest. They moved on to other areas and other toys. A lack of assertiveness was particularly evident in Johnny. No matter how intently he might be working with a puzzle or stacking a toy, he yielded it to any child who approached. Within a few weeks, however, he began shielding his activity when one of the more aggressive children approached. He used his hands and arms to push the aggressor away, even occasionally pushing the other child down and then dropping on top of him. Before long, among some of the boys, tumbling activities developed. One small car on the floor brought several interested boys. The first protected his property by lying on it, the second toppled onto the first child's body, and the next child lay across the first two. The car was forgotten as the boys rolled and tumbled together on the floor.

Mother helpers in the room took their cues from staff and learned to permit the freedom of give and take with a minimum of adult interference. For many of the children who previously had had little or no opportunity to develop peer relationships and who had been indulged by older siblings, this facet of the program opened new avenues for self-expression and socialization.

Docility was replaced with assertiveness within the classroom and even Jill, whose physical involvement was the most severe and who had appeared to be the most passive and isolated child in Group A, began to assert ownership verbally and to chastise children who approached her territory. With this assertiveness came a heightened interest in new activities and the children were quick to gather around the teacher as she demonstrated the use of a new piece of equipment or announced a variation of a group activity. Group A was indeed becoming a social entity.

This phenomenon was dramatically evidenced the day Billy returned after an absence of several weeks. He and his mother arrived after the class had started. As soon as they entered the classroom, every child broke into spontaneous applause.

CONTAGION

Early in the year when any one of the children cried, the room soon reverberated with the cries of many, if not most, of the other children. As they relaxed and lost their fear of the new surroundings, one child's tears no longer set off a chain reaction. However, it was not unusual for the staff to comment that one child's display of temper on a particular day had seemed to strike a responsive chord in several classmates, all of whom had become uncooperative or restless. By the same token, a child who entered the room filled with enthusiasm and eager to begin working often created an intensity of purpose which extended to all the classmates.

Because the children in Group B remained less socially aware, and therefore more isolated, they rarely responded to a classmate's moods, but in Group A, which reflected the blending of individual personalities into a cohesive entity, subtle differences in mood often created a general group affect. By the middle of the year the staff recognized that one child's absence or another's return would often determine the tone of that day's session.

PEER MODELING AND SOCIAL ROLES

Within the first few months two leaders emerged in Group A. Johnny and Tommy were often the first to initiate a new activity which was then imitated by the others. The two boys did not engage competitively for the role of leader but seemed to move out into the environment independent of each other.

Johnny, who enjoyed books, would go to the cupboard, select a book and sit quietly perusing it. Within minutes Melissa left her activity to choose a book and then Teresa followed suit. As the three sat on the carpet absorbed in looking at the pictures and in turning the pages, other classmates joined them in what became the library corner. When Johnny chose to paint, others in the group clamored to participate in a painting activity. Although Melissa entered the group capable of pulling herself to her feet by holding onto the table, it was Johnny who learned to grasp the top of the play stove and stand erect shortly after HEED began. Through imitation, Tommy and David learned to hold onto the stove, pulled themselves up and stood with Johnny. The staff felt that curiosity, the desire to see what Johnny was seeing, motivated Tommy and David.

Tommy led the way in initiating teasing games and in exploring. He was the first to snatch another child's cookie at the snack table. The other children learned that game quickly and soon others were engaging in it. Tommy was the first to hold onto the ledge and to stand up and look through the window into the office observation room. Each time he did this, three or four of his classmates would follow his lead and four children would peer in, tap at the window and smile and wave to the observers. When Tommy tired of the activity he left, but the other children remained, delighted with the new activity which Tommy had introduced.

When Melissa entered the program, she took toys she wanted regardless of another child's prior claim. She never shared an activity in which she displayed interest, but rather took it over. Within a few months this behavior changed somewhat. Although she still occasionally seized toys that caught her interest, she often watched a child who was having difficulty mastering a toy, moved to that child, showed him how to place the disc on the spindle, for instance, and then withdrew. In these instances she never took over the activity but seemed to be teaching by demonstration, a technique frequently employed by the teacher.

Melissa had observed the teacher at snack time placing a napkin before each child, then setting a cookie on the napkin. Soon she was replacing the napkin when a child pushed it aside or tried to use it as a toy. When a child took a bite of his cookie and then placed it on the table, Melissa replaced it neatly on the napkin.

Kate, who cried unceasingly as an outpatient in the physical therapy department and had rarely responded to the therapist's attempts to comfort her, reacted to Jill's crying by patting her shoulder and showing genuine concern for her. Kate exhibited no apprehension or anxiety for herself but seemed to be emulating the teacher in attempting to ameliorate another child's distress.

Friendships began to emerge in Group A, and parents of those children who were verbal reported that the children were talking to their families at home about their friends at school with whom they anticipated playing during the next school session. They also named the children whom they disliked. It was often impossible for the adults to pinpoint which factors engendered fondness and which behaviors elicited dislike. Some pairings lasted throughout the year and others waxed or waned from one week to the next.

EMERGENCE OF A LEADER

Antonio, who as a member of the Developmental Group had refused to separate from his mother and grandmother, both of whom accompanied him each session, exhibited the notable gains in social skills. His attachment to his mother and grandmother excluded all other contacts, staff or peer, and Antonio bellowed if anyone approached him. Because he had recently been fitted for a prosthesis and required ambulation training, the physical therapist was anxious to establish rapport with him, but Antonio rejected any overtures. Because of his obvious distress and his mother's and grandmother's indulgence, his attendance was sporadic and staff attempts to help him were unsuccessful. Finally, the team decided on full scale intervention to permit Antonio to master the separation necessary for his physical and social development. When the caseworker, who had been counseling the teenage mother, explained the staff's goals, she was able to enlist her support and the family's attendance improved. She then spoke to the grandmother who was able to admit that her protectiveness was keeping the child from achieving independent ambulation, a skill she really wished to help him acquire. With the family's cooperation the teacher then approached Antonio and told him that she was his friend and wanted to play with him. Although he immediately called her "my friend" and enjoyed using the new word, he was very cautious about relinquishing his grasp on his grandmother. Finally, with a firm admonition to play with his friend, his grandmother left the room. Although at first Antonio's howls of anger filled the room, he soon relaxed and each session he spent lengthening periods of time with the teacher and the therapist. By the time he entered HEED, he was walking independently and was secure enough to stop at the door to wave "goodbye" to his mother.

His relationships with adults were based on mutual fondness and respect, but he resisted all efforts to socialize with classmates. At home, he now competed for attention with a newborn cousin and that seemed to reinforce his dislike of his peers. When other children made advances, Antonio issued dogmatic pronouncements to any nearby adult: "He ain't my friend."

As the other children in the group began interacting with each other, the staff continued to provide inducements for Antonio to take notice of his classmates and to become friends with them.

Soon Antonio seemed to re-evaluate his position in the group and before long, he decided to assume the role of leader and entertainer. One day he firmly grasped the wooden handle of a pull toy and used it as a microphone. First, he assumed the role of a sports announcer and when he had everyone's attention, he reverted to a disc jockey and enjoined everyone: "Let's dance!" First Johnny and then a few of the other children dropped the materials with which they were involved and engaged in rhythmic rocking motions.

Within a few weeks Antonio's demeanor in the classroom changed as he set up situations to suit his own purposes. His role as a leader went unchallenged because of his verbal ability and physical prowess and his strength of will. As his third birthday approached, it was quite apparent that he was really ready for the nursery school classes where he could match his skills with children who were older and more capable of withstanding his verbal and physical onslaughts. Each session, his appearance in the HEED room was reminiscent of a maelstrom and the children accepted him not as a beloved leader, but as one who inspired awe, tinged with fear.

In the nursery school, Antonio maintains his role as one of the most verbally proficient children in his class, but he is no longer able to manipulate his peers at will and must alternate the roles of leader and follower.

THE GROUP AS A SOCIAL ENTITY

For the parents of the physically handicapped child, the differences which separate their child from others are sometimes overwhelming. Seeing the child as a reciprocal member of a social group can serve to alert the parents to future possibilities of belonging and acceptance which they had feared would be denied this particular child. The parents' awareness of the child's competence in an interactive social setting provides positive feedback for parents and reinforcement for the child. Mothers reported that the HEED youngster carried into the home songs, finger plays and social skills learned at school and sometimes became a teacher for his siblings. The flicking of the light switch to signal "clean-up time" intrigued the children and they introduced this ritual at home, to the delight of older siblings. Injunctions to sibs about "waiting your turn" surprised fathers and grandparents who viewed this development as a sign that HEED was making an impact. One mother told the parents' group that when her son taught his father "Jack in the box," the father's reservations about the program evaporated because he realized that the boy could learn to do some of the same things the older children in the family had learned at school.

Those aspects of the program which the staff discovered facilitated social awareness were having the children play side by side at the table in standing or kneeling positions, participating in activities such as clean-up time and snack time and joining in singing and rhythmic finger plays. Although the primary purpose of songs which incorporated the children's names was to produce self-awareness, they also fostered an awareness of peers and enabled the children to identify each other by name. Self-recognition was the reason for using photographs but the children's desire to look at all the pictures served as an additional means of teaching peer recognition. The staff who had not anticipated that such young children would be ready for meaningful experiences as members of a social group took their cues from the children and provided activities and opportunities for the youngsters to develop interactive social skills. The children in Group B, still involved in learning basic body mastery, required one-to-one relationships with adults, but those in Group A often outdistanced the staff in forging ahead to establish relationships with peers in a variety of roles: leader-follower, initiator-imitator, aggressor-defender. Most surprising of all was the development of eight two to three-year-olds into a cohesive social unity.

CHAPTER 11

PROMOTING COGNITIVE AND LANGUAGE LEARNING

THINKING, INTELLIGENCE, IS HIGHLY dependent upon sensory information, and upon raw material translated by the receptors and by centers in the cerebral cortex. In children who have cerebral palsy, depending upon the specific areas of the brain areas affected, decoding via one or more channels may be seriously or moderately impaired for the child. Those modalities which permit optimal cognitive functioning and promote the acquisition of conceptual thinking, inference and logic may transmit messages which are distorted or unpredictable. The distance receptors, eyes and ears, are themselves sources of incomplete or distorted environmental information for many children with cerebral palsy. Anywhere from 10 to 30 percent of cerebral palsied children are believed to have a concomitant hearing handicap, and 35 percent have involved vision (Apgar and Beck, 1972).

Difficulties in exercising voluntary control over muscles affects messages which the brain receives through various modalities, tactile and kinesthetic as well as visual. Perceptual processes, necessary precursors to cognition (Wohlwill, 1962), are estimated to be to some degrees involved in at least half of all cerebral palsied children (Apgar and Beck, 1972).

In many instances some of the problems may be at least somewhat ameliorated through surgery or corrective lenses, in the case of visual problems, or a hearing aid, in the case of hearing impairment. Therapeutic procedures, such as the relaxation of spastic muscles or the strengthening of weakened ones, through enabling the child to gain greater voluntary control over his movements, enhance the proprioceptive feedback with which he is provided by contact with his physical environment. Often, therapy takes the form of helping the child to learn to compensate for the loss of such feedback from involved areas, as in the case of learning to swallow.

In terms of special education, many of the discoveries about the properties of objects, their roundness, or hardness, for example, which are made by non-handicapped children simply through their play and the exploration with which they interact with the environment must be deliberately provided for many young children with cerebral palsy or other handicapping conditions.

DISCRIMINATING THROUGH SENSORY EXPERIENCES

The sensorial materials developed by Maria Montessori, influenced in part by the earlier pioneering work of Seguin, reflected her conviction that young children, through manipulative and repetitive use of such materials, acquired such concepts as similarity, difference, and seriation which they were subsequently able to transfer to other tasks and eventually to use abstractly in, for example, acquiring mathematical concepts. Montessori emphasized that such preconceptual skills as discrimination and classification are mastered by the child sequentially. A task requiring that form discriminations be made should not simultaneously require color discriminations until the mastery of relevant concepts had been demonstrated separately.

Whether explicitly influenced by Montessori's teaching, by inferences drawn from the writing of Piaget, or by pragmatic observation of children's apparent proclivities, nearly every nursery classroom employs concrete materials for the manipulative play of the child and a variety of activities to facilitate the learning of such concepts as form, color, number and size. Similarly, a great many commercial toys and formboard puzzles are purchased by parents, as well as nursery educators, intended to facilitate the learning of attributes of and relationships between objects.

In the HEED classroom, a variety of such materials are used, such as simple formboards and nesting toys. Each child's preference for particular materials and manner of using them are carefully observed. The degree of fine motor coordination required in the use of many such materials presents major difficulties for some children. Thus, it is necessary to consider the problem of the match from at least three perspectives: (1) the child's interest, curiosity, and exploratory propensity; (2) the child's perceptual-motor readiness, including especially fine motor coordination, and (3) the child's level of cognitive readiness for the task, e.g. his ability to solve a puzzle or place shapes in appropriate slots.

Precisely what concept the child may be learning at any given moment may be difficult to determine. Often, the teacher may observe a child at play and may sense the situation to be ripe for intervention. On one occasion, Sally had separated from the doll house the small set of stairs. Grasping one of the small wood doll figures in her hand, she proceeded to move the figure up and down the stairs. The teacher, observing this, supplied the verbal label for this action: "Up," as the doll ascended, and "Down," for the descent. After two repetitions, Sally joined in with "Up" and "Down," for the appropriate actions.

That the verbal label is not identical with the concept, but simply a means of naming it, is not disputed. Concept words, such as up, down, over, under, are considered as means of facilitating information processing. The word itself does not necessarily indicate that the concept is present. It is assumed that concepts concerning attributes of and relations between objects must be experienced, in a physical sense, by the child. Labeling cannot substitute for, but can strengthen this process.

As Sally and the teacher played with the doll and steps, Susan (prone on the floor) and Nick positioned themselves at opposite sides of the dollhouse itself. In the process of opening doors and peering through, they soon spotted each other almost simultaneously. Since each had apparently been quite engrossed in his own egocentric play, each on his respective side of the doll house, one can only guess what the significance and meaning of this discovery might have been for either. "Why Nick," said the teacher, "you can see Susan, can't you?"

A short time later, as gross motor activities elicited climbing, moving about on a large rubber ball, and crawling, Nick gleefully made for the tunnel (a cylindrical packing case with both ends removed) when the physical therapist brought it out. After making his turn through the tunnel, rapidly on all fours, Nick watched as a peer followed suit. For several more minutes he observed, still on hands and knees and still directly in the path of crawling children, almost an impediment, but undisturbed by a sensitive teacher who realized an important discovery was being made. Finally, he crawled to the opposite side and, with apparent fascination, observed the same child but from a new perspective. "Here comes Susan," said the teacher, and Nick watched Susan *going*.

The importance of avoiding overteaching, i.e. structuring every moment and every activity in a teacher-directed didactic manner, cannot be stressed too much. The adult must come to grips with his or her own definition of teaching or understanding of just what teaching means. HEED staff found that the adult role may involve diverse functions and acts. However, *observing* assumed central importance as a teaching function. Noting with what a child is engaged, his level of engagement, and what structure he seems to be imposing on the activity can inform the adult when and how she might constructively intervene. The intervention might take the form of a physical act, to slightly restructure the situation, or more commonly a verbalization, declarative or interrogative in form, which might take the form of a physical act, to slightly restructure the situation, or more commonly a verbalization, declarative or interrogative in form, which might assist the child in ordering his learning or challenging his thinking. The foregoing suggests a prior facet of the adult role: that of arranger of the environment. The discoveries made by a particular child, regardless of how serendipitous, are dependent upon an environment with which he can interact. Planning of that environment includes making available materials which may facilitate discoveries a child is ready to make, which may provide the optimal match for his evolving mental structures.

MEANS-END AWARENESS AND PERSONAL CAUSATION

"Tell me, where does a dream come from? Who makes the dreams come forth? Is it you or somebody else? Who?" Through this now familiar dialogue interview procedure, Jean Piaget sought to ascertain what sorts of explanations young children can supply for phenomena within their experience. Anyone who has engaged children in such dialogues has probably been enchanted not only with their notions but with the prelogical reasoning processes their explanations reveal.

"Is the table alive?" asks the adult.

"No," answers a five-year-old, explaining, "I never heard it talk." But the wind is alive, because "It blows." Again, the sun is more alive than a lamp, "Because it gives more light."

How do children learn to reason in this way? How and why do their reasoning processes become more logical, more veridical, more like those of adults? With the concept of egocentrism, together with the related thinking characteristics of animism, artificialism, and participation, Piaget has vividly described the reasoning characteristics of young children, as well as the developmental sequence toward more objective and relativistic explanations (Piaget, 1959; see also Ginsburg and Opper, 1969). In describing the progression from schemata, through preconcepts (Sigel, 1964), to logico-mathematical structures, he has traced the sequence leading to true hypothetico-deductive reasoning, by way of what he has called transductive reasoning, from particular to particular. Seeing one of two parallel rows of buttons, which he first regarded as equal in number, spread out and thus made longer, a four-year-old avers that it now contains more. Deceived by his perception, by the appearance of the configuration of objects, he fails to apply the principle that in order for a quantity to change, something must be added or taken away.

But the examiner (or teacher) may observe more than his error: perhaps a puzzled smile or a rather worried frown. As this child repeats the task by himself, or as he through his own spontaneous play encounters innumerable similar, but often much more personally meaningful incongruities, he is compelled to seek explanations. The *why* questions of toddlerhood, so familiar to parents, provide clues of the child's quest for explanations. That young children are untiringly engaged in a search for causal explanations, for *because's* that satisfy, through their own explorations and hypothesis testing, is well known to sensitively observant teachers.

To Piaget, the same motivating force which has enabled man to erect systems of knowledge impels the child to construct his own universe. The search for causes, the desire to know and to understand, and the need to resolve incongruity or dissonance impels the child to inquire with his actions as well as his verbalization and, like a scientist, to formulate and to test hypotheses about phenomena which are important to him.

Discovering cause-effect relationships is not a new concern for toddlers. Moving-about modes and symbol formation facilitate and provide new avenues for making such discoveries, but their roots lie in the early sensorimotor progressions of infancy. A baby cries, mother appears, and he is picked up and fed. The sequence is probably sufficiently predictable for the infant to draw inferences about causation from the correlation and temporal sequence of these events. One can observe the infant crying and looking expectantly toward the door through which his mother usually appears. As she approaches or as she lifts him from the crib, and the crying ceases as though in anticipation of what will happen next, one may infer not only that the baby has constructed a rudimentary understanding of relationships between events, but that he may have grasped a sense of the power of his own acts to bring about desired ends.

Of course such learnings do not happen spontaneously, constructed suddenly from a "buzz of confusion." They are, according to Piaget, built up sequentially and in a predictable manner.

In the course of development, children move away from absolutistic judgments and toward more relativistic ones. Naturalistic explanations come to replace magical ones. Children become increasingly able to make predictions concerning events which occur in both their physical and social environments, and consequently to experience feelings of competence concerning their own abilities to exercise rational control over such events. A child learns that it is his *act*, rather than his thought or wish, which can cause an event to occur. With experience, he learns that cause-and-effect relationships obey laws which he can generalize to new situations in the form of principles.

As Susan Isaacs has demonstrated, adults have a major role in helping young children to distinguish true causal relationships from other realities which, although important and meaningful, may often become confusing. Adult language, she believed, frequently contributes to ". . . the clouding of the child's understanding of real processes by a confusion of causal and moral categories" (1971).

> The point is well illustrated by Piaget's instance of the child who, when he was told, "You must always put a 'd' in 'grand,' " asked, "Why, what would happen if you didn't?" The child's interpretation of "must" here is surely quite logical, since he will certainly have heard the word used very often in this moral and imperative sense. And if we, in talking to children persistently use words in several different meanings, it is hardly sound psychology to attribute the whole of the resulting confusion to children's native modes of thought. This word "must," for instance, is used by adults indifferently as an assertion of will or statement of duty, as an expression of logical necessity, of invariable sequence, and of probability of inference.

The following curriculum outline relating to the generic concepts of causality, imitation, and pre-classification indicates that several interrelated areas of experience are subsumed beneath each area, each suggesting a number of specific activities. The superordinate areas, which begin to develop during the sensorimotor period, continue to evolve throughout the periods of early and middle childhood, each new learning building upon previous knowledge.

These examples of activities conducted with very young handicapped children are suggestive of a broad range, rather than comprising a prescription. Individual work with each child is characterized by an attempt to interpret observed modes of functioning in light of the framework provided by notions which are primarily Piagetian in origin. The specific activity to be undertaken at any time with any child is deter-mined more by the child's activity than by the outline. A cur-riculum outline such as this can be no more than an interpre-tive guide and coordinating center for observations and ideas generated by staff. Each child's curriculum, therefore, even given objectives in certain cognitive areas, constantly evolves.

GUIDE FOR A COGNITIVE CURRICULUM*

Flavell says that objects used by reflex patterns "perform the simple but basic function of providing grist for the activity itself, a functional sustenance which consolidates and strengthens the reflex" (Flavell, 1963). An intervention cur-riculum derived from a theory which assumes that cognitive development occurs naturally is best seen as an attempt to provide suitable grist for developing cognitive structures among children whose cognitive acquisitions have been slowed or altered by pathology.

This curriculum assumes that the general processes and rela-tionships which Piaget describes are potentially true for hand-icapped children. It seeks to use his description of stages as general diagnostic statements of cognitive capacity at a given time, and his descriptions of the transitions between stages as guides to ways of extending that capacity.

The activities in the curriculum will hopefully be interesting to children of many levels of intellectual development and available to many forms of intellectual organization. The teacher of handicapped toddlers cannot say, "Okay, we'll do this to learn that." She must interpret a given activity to each child's cognitive level and to his social and cognitive concerns. Sometimes the interpretation will involve verbal explanations; more often it will involve facilitating subsequent activity. The activities should potentially appeal to as many sensory modes as possible to enable children handicapped in one modality to compensate with another.

---

*This curriculum was developed by Mary Lou Boynton.

OBJECT PERMANENCE AND CAUSALITY

An awareness of causality depends upon the child's ability to distinguish himself and his actions from his physical world and to possess a practical spatial and temporal plan around which he can organize the interactions of persons and objects (Piaget, 1967). Mastering these relationships permits the child to escape his initial "radical unconscious egocentrism" (Piaget, 1967) and to actively pursue the environment as a source of specific satisfactions.

Causality evolves through three systems: the permanent object, temporal series, and practical space. They develop simultaneously and are interdependent. Their mutual development depends upon the child's progressing so that "early behavior becomes increasingly elaborated and differentiated to the point where the infant acquires sufficient behavioral facility for him to notice the results of his actions" (Piaget, 1967), and he becomes able to coordinate action schemata "so that some serve as a goal for action as a whole, while others serve as means" (Piaget, 1967).

A child suffering from spasticity or paralysis might be expected to have special difficulties in developing adequate sensorimotor concepts of causality. One might expect his physical world to linger in the stage of disembodied, depthless visual perceptions if he cannot reach objects to experience their solidity, or move about the room to see the many facets of familiar things, or to create "interesting effects" consistently enough to pursue them.

The techniques of physical therapy, adapted to each child and administered with an awareness of the child and his possible world, present potentially powerful cognitive tools. The "get it moving" of physical therapy applies to intelligence as well as muscles. Physical therapy equipment, such as a tire mounted on casters or sliding board, permit the child freer, more gratifying movements. A child turning on the tire sees the spatial sequence of the room and the many shapes an object assumes from different points of view. Going down the sliding board, the child can view a chair from above, at eye level, and from the bottom as he experiences the sensation of *down*. Physical therapy and its equipment, used in an environment sensitive to its cognitive potential, can assist the handicapped child to acquire the integrated experiences crucial to the development of intelligence.

The Permanent Object

The suggested activities relating specifically to object permanence are designed to encourage the child to pursue the object when it disappears, to integrate many precepts into his experience of a given object, and to use the same objects many ways. The essential goal is to fully experience an object to the end that fuller experience will reinforce a child's trust that objects do indeed exist when out of sight and away from him; they can be counted on and organized.

I. *Locating an Object in Space*

A. A bright, sound-making object is shaken within the child's visual field, the adult asking "Where's the _____?" The child is encouraged to track the object visually as it is moved at a consistent rate. The direction of movement is first horizontal, then vertical, then diagonal, then circular.

B. The above procedures are repeated, but the object is moved closer to the child so that he can grasp it. The adult can make a game of it, and respond to game-like patterns he may impose on the activity.

C. Many activities can be evolved using screens.
   1. The adult positions the child so that he faces a mirror. As he watches, the adult hides an object behind him or at his side, depending upon his attention and movement capability, and encourages him to find it.
   2. Nesting and stacking toys can be used to provide a series of screens for a hidden object. The object is

moved behind a succession of screens, gearing the number, rate of movement, and general level of difficulty to the child's observed readiness and interest.

3. Objects with distinctive shapes and textures can be wrapped in paper and the child encouraged to unwrap the package. Depending upon the developmental level of the child, the adult may encourage guessing the identity of the wrapped object.

4. A touch box challenges a child to evoke the image of an out-of-sight object. The size of the container and the aperture through which the child must reach, as well as the number and kinds of objects used, will depend upon the child's interests and successively emerging abilities.

II. Perceptual Constancy

A. The adult may present familiar objects from unfamiliar angles. She may ask for a label, or she may verbalize the relation of the aspect first seen (e.g. the legs of a doll, the wheel of a car) to the object as a whole. Or she may simply encourage the child to manipulate the object and explore it with his senses.

B. Simple puzzles provide experience in perceptual constancy by breaking a representational figure into pieces or component parts.

C. Mailbox or other shape sorter requires the child to fit a three-dimensional object into a two-dimensional space.

D. Playing with toys in sand or soapy water in which they are often partially obscured gives the child an opportunity to view isolated aspects of familiar objects.

III. Development of Multiple Schemes in Relation to an Object

A. Reversible schemes, such as folding-unfolding, crumpling-smoothing, filling-emptying, stacking-

knocking down, and manipulating play-dough can be experienced.
B. The adult may demonstrate multiple uses of object in play, such as a bead as a ball, a container as a drum, a washcloth as a blanket, or a chain as a necklace or string.
C. Often an array of toys placed before the child may share a theme.

IV. Means-end Activities

The concept of causality implies persons and things acting on each other and having a result. Means-end activities are designed to acquaint the child with the notion of *tool*. Motor patterns that have a predictable effect on the environment and objects, such as the handle of a pull toy, are all considered tools. Some areas in which the child's experiencing of means-end phenomena through tool utilization include
A. Use of knobs, as on a busy box, strings on a pull toy or other items.
B. Use of gadgets, brushes, sponges, and feathers in painting and drawing.
C. Furniture as a tool, e.g. a chair to stand on to reach a light switch.
D. Using the body as a tool
   1. Children may be encouraged to reach for things.
   2. A child with limited use of an arm can be taught to use the impaired limb to anchor paper when he draws.
   3. Carrying and arranging objects might assist a child to develop a sense of his body as a potential agent in problem solving.

V. Self and Objects in Space

Piaget traces the evolution of "practical space" from the coordination of sensory fields to a sense of the arrangement of objects and the self's relation to them: "The elaboration of

in the central area. Therapeutic techniques including naming items contained in a surprise box, manual stimulation of oral area, and impacting air were conducted by the speech pathologist with relatively homogenous groups.

Expressive language, however, permeates the learning experiences of two and three-year-old children, including those with pronounced handicaps, seriously delayed speech, and "mental-motor retardation." The expressive elements of sociodramatic play, described in Chapter 9, involve the essential features of expressive language: symbolic representation and communication. In addition, singing games and finger plays encourage vocal symbol utilization by coupling it with motoric enactment. Many of the songs suggested earlier involve simplified and repetitive actions, that is, actions such as pounding which do not represent anything other than the actions themselves, but nevertheless help to pair indicators and language.

Graphic arts media, too, can begin to be used in expressive linguistic ways. In introducing a drawing activity, the adult may point out the emptiness of the page before the child draws. After he has marked the page, the adult may show his drawing to him as an indicator of his activity. Once the basic interest in producing such effects has been aroused, and the awareness is present of the relationship between the child's intent, his action, and its effect, considerable exploration may be stimulated. The extent to which guided discovery techniques are needed will vary from child to child and from time to time. Eventually, however, the child may be able to note the relationship between the color of the crayon used and the color of the drawing.

With such a medium as finger paint, a similar procedure may be used initially, in which the child's attention will be drawn to the condition of the page prior to and during his application. He will be primarily interested here, however, in the feel of the material, and he may be encouraged to compare the way his hands feel with the feel of the painted paper. The adult may help the child to make finger and hand prints, and then to compare his own finger and hand to the images made: "See where you put your hand."

TOWARD ACQUISITION OF CONCEPTS

The basic concept-learning goals relate first to the child himself: his own body and its parts, its relation to other objects in space, and representations of himself in the form of his own name, mirror and photographic image. Necessarily, then, these goals include self-other differentiation, differentiations and similarities among other objects as preludes to classification, and most basically the concept of the permanent object.

Initial concepts of time and temporal sequence may be approached in a variety of ways. Perhaps the best examples are drawn from activities which signal that important events will immediately follow. Thus, children eagerly volunteer to flick the light switch, the signal which elicits the "It's Clean Up Time" song and appropriate activity, and chairs pushed to the table signal that snack time will follow.

Those aspects of the HEED program which relate primarily to cognitive functioning are not regarded as independent of the program as a whole. On the contrary, the program was based on recognition that children's physical, mental, social, and emotional development are not only closely interrelated, but during the first years of life, they are all of one piece, a seamless coat.

The target population comprised prime candidates for subsequent emotional and social maladjustment, ultimate school problems, and the attainment of less than an optimal quality of life during childhood, adolescence, and adulthood.

The *preventive* thrust of Project HEED was related to the presumed early needs of young children who are particularly vulnerable to disabilities associated with a primary handicapping condition of an organic nature. These disabilities can be classified at least for purposes of analysis within three major areas, corresponding to the social, emotional and cognitive spheres of development.

1. *Social:* Difficulty adjusting to social demands and feeling comfortable in social situations.

2. *Emotional:* Difficulty in achieving the birthright of human beings—a sense of effectance, competence, mastery, or au-

tonomy. This is partly related to handicaps affecting the use of physical exploration as a learning mode, and to the problem in acquiring mastery over one's own body functions. Theoretically, such difficulties suggest profound implications for the impairment of general personality development, affecting one's sense of self, or ego-identity, and attitudes and feelings toward others and toward the world.

3. *Cognitive:* Difficulty in attaining early learning during the sensorimotor period, learning which involves the successive coordination and integration of sensory and motor schemas, or action patterns. Such handicaps may impair acquisition of important building blocks of intelligence, including the concept of the permanent object; body orientation in space; imitation, and causality. These are needed for acquisition of concepts *about* objects, for inferential reasoning, for hypothesis formation and testing, for modeling and for deferred imitation, which leads also to the development of imagination. It is not clear theoretically how essential the role of language functions is in the attainment of symbolic functioning. It is very clear, however, that a great many handicapped children evidence uneven, delayed, or disturbed language development.

CHAPTER 12

CONSIDERATIONS AND APPROACHES IN BEHAVIOR MANAGEMENT

CONSISTENCY IN MANAGEMENT provides all children with the security of knowing the limits imposed. With the neurologically handicapped, consistency is probably of greater importance in helping the child to structure his environment. Impulsive behavior and the inability to employ inhibiting restraints often characterize the brain damaged child. Limits must be set by the adult and systematically and consistently enforced if the child is to be helped to understand what behavior is expected of him and what behavior will not be permitted. Because the hyperkinetic child often is consumed with guilt after he has caused injury to a peer or an adult, he welcomes firm consistent limits.

An example illustrating the validity of this principle even with very young children is provided by the following anecdote. Gerald, age three, upon meeting the project director, quickly snatched her glasses. She took the glasses from Gerald and as she replaced them, Gerald reached to repeat the act. A firm "No" and a hand placed quickly over his stopped him. Moments later he snuggled on her lap as she sat on the floor taking part in a group activity. It was the staff's belief that Gerald was relieved and grateful for the external restraint which she had provided for him.

To have explained to Gerald at that time the reasons for not pulling off the glasses would have served little purpose. What was needed was a prompt firm response to stop him from an unacceptable impulse, to communicate a clear simple message, as well as to prevent the destruction of the glasses. Later, when he greeted the adult with a hug and then gazed solemnly at her glasses, she explained that she needed to wear them so that she could see.

He became more aware of body involvement and was frustrated by the limits imposed by his involved hand.

However, with the increased alertness appeared a great deal of aggressive acting out, mainly in the form of hitting. Gerald appeared a very angry child, and his mother freely expressed her inability to cope either with his behavior or with her own feelings of counter-aggression and desperation. Her need simply to unburden herself of her feelings was so great that she was eager to share these problems and was actively reaching out for help, for herself as well as for Gerald.

During her first interview with an agency caseworker, Gerald was characteristically disruptive and made conversation impossible. However, though his mother became increasingly distraught, she seemed unable to intervene effectively. Noting this, the caseworker rose from her seat, said, "Do you mind if I try?" and, in a kind but firm manner, took Gerald by the hand and led him to a small table in the office on which were play materials, saw to it that he became occupied with these, and returned to her chair. "How did you do that?" asked the startled mother, which led into a discussion of child management. For some time thereafter, whenever this mother described how helpful the HEED program had been to her personally, as well as to her child, she illustrated with this episode.

This confusion about a child's problems in accepting limits, and in the distinction between limiting behavior and punitiveness, presented a major problem for many parents. In Gerald's case, upon his entrance into the HEED program, his initial behavior was characterized by striking out at all who came near him and by aimless wandering about the room and into the hall. The teacher's assistant was assigned to work with him in a constant one-to-one relationship in order to provide both relationship and consistent controls. After a few sessions of resistance, he came rapidly to accept her, and soon thereafter transferred his trust to the teacher and physical therapist.

LEARNING THROUGH STRUCTURE

The concept of structure implies order, predictability, and boundaries. Humans can be observed to impose structure upon their environment and experiences in a variety of ways, as well as to respond to structure which has been externally imposed.

Those who work with young children attempt to organize learning experiences along the dimensions of time and space in ways which will enable children more readily to impose their own organization.

Some elements of structure in the HEED program intended to foster ego development and positive social interaction relate to the scheduling of activities, others to arrangement of the physical environment, and still others to specific behaviors of adult staff members. Actually, the general situation itself, a peer group classroom setting with several adults present, establishes some parameters, dictates certain roles, and creates behavioral expectations which serve to structure what will and what will not take place.

Many learning programs for exceptional children, including mildly neurologically impaired or otherwise hyperactive or distractible children, as well as more seriously handicapped, attempt to create a stable and predictable sequence. Each day, certain events take place in an established order so that children can both experience security through sameness and routine and be able to predict events, thus gaining cognitively. With young multiply handicapped children, familiarity must precede discovery. Knowing what will happen next provides the child with a necessary sense of psychological safety which enables him to anticipate events and to initiate behavior in light of his predictions.

HEED children appear to internalize classroom routines very readily: clean-up time precedes use of the slide, large ball and other large muscle equipment; removal of these items signals that snack time is next, and many children soon come to move spontaneously toward the chairs which must be pushed over to the table. Climbing into their chairs, some children begin to "clap, clap your hands" in anticipation of the singing game. As some children ask for *more* juice or cookie, one or two children will look toward the door through which mother will soon enter.

As the children are finishing snack, the teacher's assistant takes books from the cupboard and places them on the carpet. Many children quickly finish the last morsel of cookie and head for the carpet. The action of the teacher's assistant often serves to provide the needed cue for the dawdlers, since they appear to anticipate the next sequence.

Often the children's eyes move from the pictures in the book to the doorway and, as soon as the teacher suggests "Let's call Mommy," children begin moving toward the door to call their mothers who are in the kitchen at the top of the stairs.

The principles of environmental influences on the structuring of behavior sequences are derived from diverse sources. The Montessori classroom is regarded as a structured learning environment, but the Montessori pedagogy illustrates a principle often overlooked by educators. To some, *structure* may imply a high degree of directive adult control, possibly repressive control. In the Montessori classroom, structure is inherent in the physical setting itself, including the specific physical materials of which it is comprised. Reinforcement theorists, too, establish as a general principle that behavior is sustained or altered by contingencies in the environment. The adult's role is that of providing opportunities for and monitoring the interaction of child and environment.

LEARNING ABOUT CONSEQUENCES

A useful rule asserted by advocates of contingency management or behavior modification approaches, with children and adults, is that behavior is maintained by its consequences. If a behavior is emitted with relative consistency, it can be assumed that something in the environment is reinforcing that behavior. This position has it that, beyond elemental reflexes, all behavior is learned, that is, it is acquired through interaction with the environment, from which differential patterns of reinforcement serve to shape one's repertoire of response dispositions.

The applications of this view to teaching and various forms of therapeutic intervention are obvious. First, one must observe systematically in order to determine precisely what behaviors are occurring and with what frequence. The teacher or therapist can then set about to modify a behavioral pattern through attempting to arrive at the right combination of reinforcer and schedule of reinforcement. Applications range from the fairly unsystematic systems of reward used by most parents and teachers to highly systematized token economies. Where careful and thorough procedures of observation and experimental analysis of specified behaviors have been employed, desirable results have characteristically been reported. The system "works" in terms of the elimination of undesirable behaviors and, more importantly, the shaping of desirable ones.

Unfortunately, critical discussions of behavior modification too often degenerate into diatribes on the evils of mind control, cold efficiency in the management of human beings, denial of human volition, and the like. The point made by proponents of behavior modification through operant conditioning principles is not so much that behavior *can* or *should* be controlled by environmental contingencies; rather, that it *is* so controlled.

The degree to which an individual is consciously aware of the consequences of a particular action varies from situation to situation and certainly from individual to individual. If one can be said to be controlled by the consequences of his acts upon the environment, that is, by what effects of these actions are fed back to him, this is not to say that one cannot learn to influence the flow of environmental feedback he receives simply by exerting cognitive control over his actions. A child can learn to predict what the consequences of particular actions may be. He can become aware of cause-effect relationships, particularly those involving his own behavior.

The theoretical perspective and experimental observations of Piaget place great stress on such learning of causal relationships. The concepts of *effectance motivation* and *sense of competence*, advanced by Robert White, relate the subjective aspects of ego-enhancement to motivation and learning in the causal area. In terms of the acquistion of prosocial behavior, or learning to regulate one's own activity as a participant in a social milieu, causal thinking has long been stressed in the writing of Ralph Ojemann (see, for example, Ojemann, 1961). The ability to predict what will occur as a consequence of any of several alternative courses of action enables an individual to select from among alternatives, to mediate both external constraints and internal impulses, and to exert rational control over his own behavior.

Eli Bower has described the increased range of response alternatives to a given situation in terms of "degrees of freedom" (Bower, 1967). For example, a small child can, when thwarted, resort to comparatively few avenues, perhaps having a tantrum or some form of withdrawal from the situation. An older child can, however, employ verbal argument, choose another compromise goal, or apply subtle forms of manipulation known well by parents.

A major aspect of behavior is, therefore, the acquisition of abilities to predict what will happen as a consequence of behavior, and of the realization that desirable or aversive consequences to oneself are not random events. Consistency in management, traditionally advocated if not always practiced on the basis of intuition and common sense, finds greater support from the standpoint of both reinforcement and cognitive-competence views.

In work with young multiply handicapped children, however, some situations arise which suggest that consistency and consequence-oriented management may be difficult to effect, if not at time contraindicated. For example, David had demonstrated the ability to use appropriately several words, among them "more" when desiring additional milk or cookies at snack time. However, for a time, he was inconsistent in supplying the verbalization, often extending his cup or hand and otherwise indicating his desire, but not using the word *more* or the expression *more milk* or *more cookie*. In the interest both of maintaining his expressive repertoire and of encouraging him to use appropriate social behavior, the staff debated the merits of withholding the item until he produced the word. It was suggested that the teacher might ignore him until the word was forthcoming.

However, other considerations were raised. David had demonstrated his competence relative to these words. Would insistence on their utterance represent a concern for mechanical performance at the expense of more basic goals, such as security and pleasure in the group setting? Furthermore, David continued to demonstrate good progress in his acquisition of expressive vocabulary and use of speech in classroom activity. The fear that his expressive vocabulary would atrophy through disuse seemed ill-founded. Further, the teacher observed that David frequently had difficulty in organizing his thoughts in this and other situations. It was known that David had a central processing disturbance, and it was suspected that he was having frequent petit mal seizures. The staff concluded that to withdraw reward would be punitive. Rather than to ignore his poorly formed request pending emission of the verbalization, it was determined to capitalize on these incidents as opportunities to help David form his intent. For one thing, the pace at which second helpings were dispensed appeared somewhat too rapid for David. It was determined that the teacher would attend to any signal from David, smile and wait, supply encouragement and cues, and respond to approximations to the desired verbalization with the desired milk or cookie.

It is occasionally not clear that the reason an adult intervention is effective is that the child is aware that attainment of a desired reward is contingent upon complying with an adult request. One day the gross motor session involved the use of chairs, barrel, and steps, set up as an obstacle course. The children were delighted with the new activity and joined in with glee. Kate, however, feigned fear and resisted participating. The teacher, who was across the room near the door, reminded Kate it was her turn to get the cookies for snack and Kate came quickly to the teacher by way of the obstacle course, maneuvering with surprising agility and with no semblance of fear. Staff were uncertain whether Kate had recognized the relationship between her participation in the activity and the desired event, a relationship only implied, not stated explicitly, by the teacher. The salient element may have been the child's momentary diversion. Or it may have been her sense of the teacher's expectations regarding her behavior.

Relative to these latter elements, another incident provides an illustration of noncoercive, yet firm and effective management. At the conclusion of a session several children refused to relinquish the small cars they were holding. Mothers scolded and attempted to pry the toys from clenched fingers. A staff member picked up an empty box and went to each child saying, "Drop the car here," and everyone complied. Perhaps the box was a diversion and served to turn the confrontation into a game, but the firm voice of an adult who expected compliance also served to remind the children that within the classroom there are limits which they are expected to know and to accept.

Sometimes, however, firmness may lead to confrontation, and diversion may bring about more readily the desired goal. Melissa's mother often expressed an inability to cope with Melissa when she "pitched a fit" out of sheer "stubbornness." Insistence on Melissa's holding an adult's hand to practice walking brought immediate resistance and a temper tantrum. The physical therapist utilized a monkey hand puppet to encourage Melissa to walk when the child refused to hold the therapist's hand. Holding the thumb of the therapist's hand, which was encased in the puppet, was acceptable to Melissa, and before long she was walking happily throughout the building holding the monkey's hand as the physical therapist gradually removed her own fingers until Melissa was walking independently.

LEARNING ABOUT FEELINGS

Gaining a degree of cognitive control over one's emotions is probably dependent in large part on language, on having words for the feelings. A child's strong emotion, such as anger or fear, can be frightening to him. The technique of supplying to the child the word for the way he feels conveys that the emotion has a name and that others understand what he is feeling. In working with very young children, many of whom are still pre-lingual, however, the technique of verbalization may be more difficult to employ to the same advantage.

One illustration of the applicability of verbalization is provided in the instance of separation of mother from child. A mother must often be encouraged to allow her child the opportunity to experience the feeling of grief or anxiety and to express it. Sometimes a mother will be unable to leave if the child cries. The readiness of the child for this separation must be gauged. The teacher may say, "You miss your mother, but she'll be right back." This can reassure the child that his mother will return, but it also conveys that his concern is legitimate and is understood. Mothers are urged to say, "I'm going upstairs to get a cup of coffee," rather than attempt to slip out unnoticed. Words can come to be very powerful tools in sorting out the complexities of what would otherwise be random and anxiety inducing events.

When a child cries because he has fallen or bumped his head, the teacher holds him, gently massages the affected part and supplies the words, "I know it hurts." A combination of holding and talking to the child reassures him that he is cared for and cared about. Never is he told that he has no reason to cry. The words "it hurts" let him know that someone understands his pain.

When a piece of equipment new to Kate was introduced into the room, Kate evidenced panic by crying. The teacher immediately assured her that she need not take part in the activity. With her arm around the child the teacher encouraged her to observe the other children crawling through the barrel and pointed out, "You see the barrel doesn't hurt Billy. He's having fun." But under no circumstances would the adult deny Kate's fear about the equipment. When the mother of a newly enrolled child entered the classroom, Tommy recoiled in fear and the teacher placed herself near him and promised that she would stay close by because "You don't know Teresa's Mommy and that makes you afraid." In very simple language which Tommy could understand the teacher told him that when he did get to know the new Mommy, he would no longer be fearful.

Terry was unaccustomed to peers and was docile and unassertive when she entered. Johnny found her to be fair prey and delighted in grabbing a toy from her. Terry's screams of anger and frustration increased Johnny's pleasure in the one-sided game. The teacher verbalized Terry's anger and encouraged her to say, "No! That's mine." She also encouraged her to hold on to her possession tightly. Thus, Terry learned from the teacher that it was acceptable to be angry with Johnny and more important, perhaps, that it was acceptable to assert herself in protecting what was rightfully hers.

When a class is clapping hands during a rhythmic activity, the joy in participating in a rhythmic activity brings smiles and wiggles. The teacher imitates by swaying and smiling and thus enters into the child's enjoyment and pleasure. Words in this instance are unnecessary in responding to the child's emotion. Whether it be by verbalizing the child's feelings, by supplying the appropriate word, or by comforting him through one's presence, the child is made aware that someone both understands and respects his feelings.

SUPPORT AND GUIDANCE FOR PARENTS

It has repeatedly been stressed that many parents of young handicapped children experience unusual problems in the management of their children's social behavior. On the one hand, the child's handicap itself may present barriers to the acquisition of desirable social behaviors. A child who is hemophilic or has brittle skeletal structures may be protected from encounters with the instructive realities of the physical environment, through which children can learn to temper impulses in deference to the Freudian reality principle.

For motorically impaired children, restricted physical exploration may have the same consequence. Parents may to varying degrees be able to allow their child to have these experiences, but it may often be far easier to carry the child, to bring a toy to him, to feed him, and in general to create a system of mutual expectancies not conducive to the growth of responsibility and social consideration.

On the other hand, it is a rare parent who can respond to his or her child without a degree of ambivalence or conflict, especially if the child is handicapped. Parental guilt may lead to nonintervention and inability to exert needed controls and

guidance, thus tacitly encouraging tyrannical or hedonistic behavior. Parents of handicapped children, too, often experience
a sense of bondage. Neither martyrdom nor suppressed and
controlled anger is conducive to healthy parent-child relations.
Often the sheer stress of coping with a child's physical needs
may leave little psychic energy left over for dealing sensitively
with emotional needs and behavioral guidance. Often, too, the
label *exceptional* may color even a parent's expectancies toward
the child, so that the basic fact that he is first of all a child may
be, in some ways, overlooked.

The models provided by staff members may be helpful to
parents who observe the classroom interaction setting or participate in it. Indeed, HEED parents with few exceptions have
indentified their learning from professional staff, both through
counsel and example, as one of the most valuable facets of the
program.

A mother may also gain insight into the whys of a technique
used by a staff member. In some areas a mother-child relationship deteriorates into a series of confrontations in which the
mother finds herself arguing and the child resisting until the
mother in frustration overcomes the impasse by sheer physical
force. Her feelings of guilt and inadequacy then plague her to
the extent that she relinquishes that role and permits the child
to manipulate her. However, this new role is anger producing
and many mothers have expressed their confusion and chagrin
at having lost control in the area of behavior management.

The staff member is, of course, able to respond somewhat
more objectively to a child's behavior, hopefully not in conflict
concerning her own role, expectancies, or feelings toward the
child. It is much easier to cope with insistent whining and
refusal when one does not need to do so much of the day, day
after day, month after month.

Often a parent expresses, or suggests through what is not
said, a sense of inadequacy upon seeing how well the teacher or
therapist may handle situations with which she herself finds it
difficult to cope. At such times the parent is assured that the
problems she faces are difficult indeed, that managing the child
in the program setting presents in many ways an ideal situation,

in contrast to those which occur at home. She is urged, however, to analyze with the staff member, usually the caseworker, what it was that *was* done, why the teacher's handling of a situation was effective, and how she might be able to apply any of the principles which the incident might have illustrated.

Often such discussions take place between parents, either informally in conversation or in a parent group meeting. It is important to clarify that there is no simple formula to apply in child management, and certainly no magic. The observation experience serves to take the parent out of the conflict situation, in which her own needs and defenses may play a greater role than she realizes. From the vantage point of an observer, the parent may see her child and one of his typical behavior patterns in a new light. Such new insights provide much material for guidance by staff members, for supportive casework, and for parent group discussions around mutual problems.

CHAPTER 13

CASE STUDIES OF REPRESENTATIVE CHILDREN

T HE THREE CHILDREN WHO HAVE been chosen for the following case studies are representative of other children in the program insofar as their diagnoses, experiences in HEED, progress noted during the year and future educational planning are concerned. The blend of these elements along with other experiential and attitudinal factors created a unique situation for each child and each family; therefore, all teaching and therapy procedures, as well as counseling and future educational planning were individualized to accommodate each specific child and family.

Nick's neurological involvement caused delayed responses to stimuli and created an unevenness of achievement. He is typical of the largest number of children in the program. Peter was representative of those children whose mental retardation was their most severe impairment. Teresa's physical disorder seemed to be limiting insofar as independent ambulation was concerned but did not interfere with manual dexterity or cognitive ability. Thus, these children, although given the individuality of each specific situation, serve to portray three distinct patterns representative of HEED children.

NICK: A CASE STUDY

Early Development and Medical History

Nick is the only child of parents in their late twenties. He was born ten weeks prematurely and remained in an incubator for four weeks. Shortly after his release from the hospital, his mother noted an inflexibility in his legs when she diapered him.

When he was one year old, the pediatrician suggested a diagnostic evaluation in a hospital program which the parents discovered was no longer in operation. No further diagnostic referral was made at that time. The mother was concerned about Nick's delayed language and motor development and the family initiated a single contact with a hearing and speech clinic when Nick was twenty months of age. At that time the parents were informed that the child appeared to be functioning at a fifteen month level in terms of language and personal-social behaviors. The therapist's report noted that the mother, although fearful because of her younger brother's diagnosis of cerebral palsy, was using child rearing practices which were both realistic and appropriate for Nick's functional age. When Nick was two years old, a referral was made to an orthopedist who diagnosed minimal brain damage, and prescribed physical therapy at the Society for Crippled Children where Nick received weekly treatment for three months.

HEED Participation

In January, 1973, when Nick was two years and four months of age, he entered HEED. In the initial series of evaluations and assessments administered he achieved the following scores:

Cattell Infant Intelligence Scale	21.5 months
Vineland Social Maturity Scale	20 months
Preschool Attainment Record	23 months
Physical Therapy	12 months
Occupational Therapy	21 months
Houston Test for Language Development	6 months
Bzoch-League Receptive-Expressive Emergent Language Scale	21 months

Nick was a blond robust child who smiled frequently and exhibited minimal anxiety in the new situation. During the first few sessions he explored the classroom, manipulated the toys and responded to the teacher by smiling shyly. The second week after entry he was able to separate from his mother with no indication of distress when she left the room.

By the end of the first month he showed an increased awareness of the other children and was completely comfortable with
the teacher and therapists. He was especially intrigued with the
small cars and trucks and whenever the child size car was
available, he climbed onto it, made engine sounds and swayed
back and forth as though he were maneuvering corners. Although he had initially rejected all table tasks requiring manual
dexterity, he was amenable to direction and soon learned to
match shapes and to complete simple puzzles. He initiated play
with the pegs and on the formboard and often spent as long as
fifteen minutes in deep concentration, rarely seeking assistance, as he engaged himself in problem solving tasks.

Although Nick was not walking, he engaged in all areas of
gross motor activity with great enjoyment. His standing balance
improved and he was able to knee-walk with the support of a
chair which he pushed. He was encouraged to stand for water
play and table activities, but he tended to stand up on his toes
with hips and knees flexed. His left leg appeared slightly more
involved than the right, and this made ambulation difficult
because it was hard for him to step forward with the left leg and
to place his heel on the floor. However, his crawling pattern
was good, and he continued to participate in gross motor activities with glee and abandon.

He responded without visual clues to simple directions such
as "Take your chair to the table" or "Push the wagon." His
expressive language increased in the classroom and he was
communicating his needs, addressing peers and answering
questions with single word responses. His mother had reported
a larger repertoire of words a few months earlier, words which
he seemed to have dropped. A referral for an audiological
evaluation was made by the speech pathologist who viewed his
transient vocabulary and word loss as an indication of a possible
problem of hearing acuity. The audiometric evaluation, accomplished without the use of earphones because of Nick's
resistance, revealed borderline to normal limit hearing and a
recommendation was made for a re-evaluation in six months to
determine the status of each ear.

As Nick's interest in his peers and in the materials and

equipment available expanded, his play became more creative and social skills emerged. When Gerald was summoned to turn off the lights, Nick quickly brought him a chair to stand on. He exchanged toys with the other children and he offered another child the toy with which he had just finished playing. He had always permitted children to take toys from him without demur; by April he was crying when a toy was taken from him, but he still lacked assertiveness in defending his property rights. He intently observed the activities of his classmates and reacted to their enjoyment by smiling broadly and hurrying across the room to join them.

During finger play and singing activities which preceded snack, Nick's expression was one of total absorption as he leaned forward to watch and listen. When he was ready to join, his body relaxed, his hands performed the gestures, and he sang the words with gusto. At first it appeared that this child needed to master a situation internally to acquire confidence in its performance. But his ultimate participation was always one or two steps behind the group. As the teacher and children chanted "Tap, tap, tap the table," Nick was engaged in the words and gestures from the preceding verse, even with those songs and rhythms which were repeated each session. In a review of the day's events members of the staff often commented that Nick seemed slow in processing information, but that his learning potential appeared adequate.

In April a note in the Teacher's Daily Record reported that Nick did not seem to understand the teacher, that he maintained eye contact but exhibited a "blank look." Throughout May the teacher continued to report that Nick sometimes did not understand a direction or a routine he had understood and responded to before. Although he still remained a generally physically active youngster, he was now spending part of almost every session in passive positions, e.g. sitting at the table with head bowed or in the car unmoving and unresponsive to invitations to join in activities. Fears arose in areas where none had been exhibited before. He clung to his mother and refused to let her leave him. The fears extended to equipment and materials he had used freely and had thoroughly enjoyed such as the slide and tricycle. Usually the teacher was able to reassure him and he derived comfort from a short ride in the wagon or on the swing and then was able to resume his usual play habits. His mother reported another element in his life which might be creating distress. The family's improved finances enabled the parents to engage in more evening social experiences and Nick was unhappy about being left with a babysitter. As the weather improved, part of each day was spent out of doors and it seemed possible that the change of environment had induced anxiety which led to the fearful and withdrawn behavior. Another possible explanation was that the delayed separation anxiety was consistent with Nick's general behavioral pattern.

In June his need for his mother's immediate presence lessened, but he preferred to have her near by, either in the observation room where he could glance up and see her or somewhere in the classroom or on the playground so that she could smile and wave when he showed her a toy and called "Look, Mom." He was able to permit her to leave but if she did not return within half an hour, he occasionally interrupted his play to look toward the door with some anxiety. He was usually comforted by the teacher's explanation that his mother was having a cup of coffee in the kitchen or talking to someone in the office. Before long, he transferred his dependence on his mother to a more independent relationship with the staff.

Nick continued to make gains in language and in problem solving activities. He would choose the more complex materials and would often work for as long as twenty minutes on mastering one task. When he was unable to manage one step of the several required to unscrew the handle of a spindle, remove the discs and then replace the discs and handle, he took the spindle to the teacher and solicited her help by placing her hand on the handle. He then returned to the task and persisted through a trial and error approach until he had mastered all of the steps required. In fact, he discovered that by removing the knobs at either end he could freely slide the discs on and off, and he impishly demonstrated this new use. He finished by replacing knobs and discs with no further help. The entire procedure lasted for approximately half an hour. His mother reported that at home he was learning to open and close caps of jars and bottles. She said he rarely requested help but preferred to "work things out for himself." Her pride in his persistence and independence was obvious.

At home he was beginning to speak in short sentences; at school two word phrases were heard more frequently during May and June.

Although Nick's progress in social, cognitive and language development was steady, his pattern of delayed response and his brief periods of loss of contact with the environment continued to concern the staff and his mother.

When the evaluations which had been administered in January were repeated in July, Nick showed gains in all areas. A four month gain was noted in speech and in unilateral and bilateral skills. He had also improved in self-care skills. The educational evaluation showed marked gains in self-awareness, purposive play and social interaction with peers and adults. The psychological evaluation showed a strengthening of verbal skills and greater persistence in working with objects. Only in the area of gross motor functioning, as determined by means of a physical therapy diagnostic assessment, was there a lack of significant progress. Figure 13-1 shows the comparative results of evaluations administered in January, July and December.

The program resumed in September following a four week vacation. On his return, Nick appeared to have consolidated the gains noted. Along with four classmates, he began to visit the Agency nursey school for short periods of time every week. These five were the HEED children for whom plans were being formulated for entrance into the regular nursery school classes some time after the first of the year. Nick enjoyed the visits but wanted his teacher to remain close by. He enjoyed the creative projects in the nursery school and became engrossed in them. He soon became comfortable with the nursery school teachers and was able to separate from HEED staff.

Along with an increased ability to respond to his environment and to interact with peers and adults there still existed intermittent periods of loss of contact and loss of acquired skills. This created an unevenness in performance and in af-

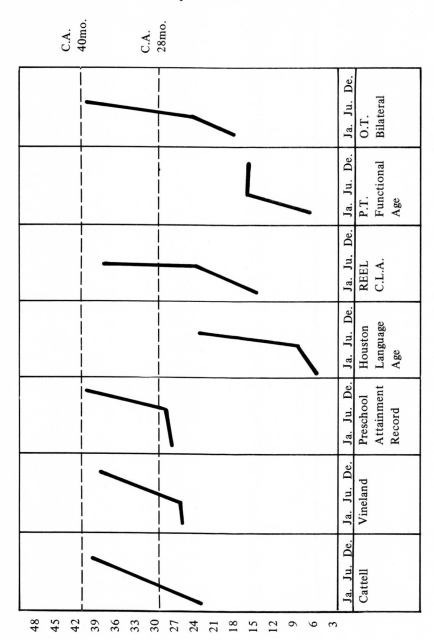

fect. For example, on the same day that he used scissors appropriately he was unable to replace large round pegs. In staffing sessions shared observations led to the conclusion that the "tuning out" phenomenon seemed at least partially associated with excessive verbal input and changes in the environment such as moving the class outdoors. But the diagnosis of brain damage raised the question of possible petit mal episodes. Nick's glazed expression often interrupted a task in which he was completely involved and was followed by immediate resumption of the task.

Nick's parents shared the staff's concern and agreed to seek a complete neurological evaluation. A referral was made to a pediatric comprehensive care unit of a local hospital. No substantially new findings were discovered, and after his discharge from the hospital, Nick and his mother returned to the HEED program.

Parents

Because Nick's mother was able to express her own and her husband's concerns and insights, her role as an integral member of the team was quickly established. She participated freely in discussions as problems arose and in decisions as solutions were sought. Her agreement with the philosophy and goals of the program and the strategies employed to attain those goals, as well as her ability to interpret them to her husband, enabled the parents to expand the program into a total life experience for their son. Camping trips and related outdoor ventures, cooking and baking opportunities enriched Nick's life and extended his education and rehabilitation beyond the boundaries of the class-room.

The mother reported that her own depression activated by her son's delayed development began to dissipate within the first six weeks after entering into HEED. Her need for contact with adults was met by her association with the mothers in the group, and her need to understand her son's development was fulfilled by her contacts with the staff. One can speculate that her basic loneliness, akin to that of many young mothers whose days are spent apart from other adults, was compounded by anxieties about her son.

Although her husband had always maintained an active involvement in Nick's medical progress during the HEED experience, she described the quality of the father-son relationship as improved. The boy began to emerge as more "interesting" because he was "doing more." Nick's mother indicated that the marked change which occurred in her with the easing of her apprehension may also have been responsible for the improvement in the relationship of Nick and his father.

The mother often took notes during the parent session when the teacher or a therapist addressed the group to refresh her memory when she shared the information on therapy or educational techniques with her husband. And when he desired additional clarification on a staff recommendation, he took time from work to visit and to confer with members of the staff. It was apparent that both parents were actively involved in the child rearing process.

Although during the initial in-take interview Project HEED had been explained to her in detail, Nick's mother confided at the end of the year that she had not anticipated what for her had been the most rewarding aspects of the program. The informality of the exchanges with the professional staff and her acceptance as a partner on the team were the factors which she felt enabled her to voice her fears and to participate optimally in the staff's efforts on behalf of herself and her child.

The relationships in Nick's family, although basically warm and loving, had been strained by the parents' fears and doubts about their son's medical diagnosis and his future. The HEED experience served to heighten their understanding of Nick's development and to enhance their parenting skills.

Summary

At the conclusion of a year in the HEED program, Nick's hip stability and standing balance were improved, he could knee-walk and he had progressed in independent standing for brief periods. He displayed interest in assisting in dressing and undressing himself. He was communicating with teachers and classmates in phrases and simple sentences. The teacher reported increasing self-awareness and a continually expanding interest in new materials and activities.

In January, 1974, Nick entered the agency nursery school. He enjoyed the new experience of riding on the school bus and although his mother accompanied him for the first week, he was comfortable and secure enough in the new setting to permit her to remain in the observation room. When he entered the locker room, on his first day, he recognized the photographs of children who had been his classmates in the HEED program, and he spontaneously pointed to each picture and supplied the correct name. His teachers report that he is an active and eager participant in all areas of the nursery school program.

PETER: A CASE STUDY

Early Development and Medical History

Peter is the fourth of five children, the two oldest of whom are adopted. The mother had had periods of bleeding during the pregnancy and had received hormone shots. The delivery was uneventful, and there was no mention of birth anomalies, but at three months of age Peter developed pneumonia and was treated with medication which the mother reports was subsequently withdrawn from the market. After his recovery, his mother became concerned about his slow development. A spinal tap revealed a protein deficiency. The mother also reported that at that age Peter seemed "flabby and lethargic," and was unable to sit unassisted. The pediatrician referred the family to a pediatric neurologist who hospitalized the child for further evaluation. Questions were raised concerning etiology of symptoms and the possibility of a genetic disorder or of vitamin B deficiency. The diagnosis which emerged from the test findings was motor retardation and brain disorder. The mother who was convinced that the medication administered when Peter was an infant was responsible for the damage, disagreed with the physician's conclusion that Peter's condition was present at birth.

When Peter was twenty-seven months old, a referral for physical therapy was made to the Society for Crippled Children. The initial therapy evaluation in June, 1971 indicated that Peter was a good-sized one-year-old with fair head control. His lower extremities exhibited some tension; the upper extremities were floppy. He had no sitting balance and although he could lift his head, he could hold it up for only a few seconds when he was placed on his stomach. He was scheduled for weekly appointments, and a home program was planned to strive for head control, sitting balance and head and arm use from the prone position. Five months later, the therapist noted that head control was good, sitting balance had improved, but that Peter tended to lean forward on his arms when seated with legs extended.

Developmental Play Group

Peter entered the Developmental Play Group, forerunner of HEED, in September, 1972, when he was two and one-half years old. He could not separate from his mother and cried uncontrollably when she was not directly in view. His sitting balance was precarious and he had poor head and trunk stability. While sitting on the floor he often threw himself backward. The only objects he exhibited any interest in manipulating were the ball and a wad of facial tissues.

His mother who was in the fourth month of pregnancy often commented wryly, "Peter had better shape up before the baby comes!"

Heed Participation

In January, 1973, Peter was enrolled in HEED. Although he was now coming into a new classroom, he was comfortable in the setting. He smiled at the staff with recognition and was willing to separate from his mother.

The following are the results of Peter's initial evaluation:

Cattell Infant Intelligence Scale	10 months
Vineland Social Maturity Scale	8 months
Preschool Attainment Record	11 months
Physical Therapy	4 months
Occupational Therapy	9 months
Houston Test for Language Development	5 months
Bzoch-League Receptive-Expressive Emergent Language Scale	5.5 months

Peter was a chubby genial child who responded to the teacher and the therapist with vocalizations and smiles. His sitting balance had improved during the past few months but he was still unable to sit unaided. When he was on his stomach, he showed awareness of toys placed in front of him, but he could not pull himself along the floor to reach them.

His interest in toys remained limited but the rice mixture attracted his attention. When he was seated on the floor with the pan of rice between his legs, he handled the mixture cautiously at first, then ventured to place both hands into the rice and finally he used his hand to throw the rice out of the container. This repetitive motion seemed to bring him great pleasure.

By the end of January Peter used fewer random hand and arm motions in reaching and grasping. He was able to pick up a bowl that was upside down and to replace it right side up. As Peter became more aware of his surroundings, the teacher noted in her daily report that the environment was serving to stimulate and enrich Peter's development.

An indication of his increased awareness was the uneasiness he exhibited when an unfamiliar adult entered the classroom. Previously, he had seemed oblivious of the presence of the other children, but he was now viewing them as a threat to himself and his toy and would grasp their hair if they approached him when he was engaged in playing with the rice, for example. Although he was unable to imitate simple gestures, when a member of the staff played pat-a-cake or peek-a-boo, he grinned and shook his hands up and down excitedly.

In mid-January, Peter moved six inches unaided along the floor to retrieve a cup he had thrown. To allow him greater experience of movement, the physical therapist placed him on a scooter board. He overcame his fear of the scooter board within a few sessions and by mid-March was able to move around the room for short distances on the scooter board. This increased mobility signalled an increased awareness of other toys available. He would pick up one object, transfer it to his other hand, pick up another and then hit the two objects together.

Peter's baby sister was born in February, and for approximately four weeks he was accompanied to class by his father. There seemed to be little significant change in Peter's behavior during this time. But by the end of March he became irritable, cried and fussed for no apparent reason and would not be comforted, even by his mother who was now coming with him and bringing the infant. Periods of crying and whining were interspersed with apathy. The behavior was so unlike Peter that discussions of this behavior ensued with mother and staff. The mother reported that since the baby's birth Peter was not being handled as much as he had been, and it seemed quite likely that he was unhappy about having been replaced as the baby in the family. During the HEED sessions the baby usually slept quietly either in the observation room or in the kitchen, but the staff wondered if Peter felt that class time belonged to him and his mother and resented the baby's presence in an area that he viewed as his own.

Because the baby was breast fed and also because of the difficulty in making arrangements, it was not always possible for the infant to be left at home. But the mother did manage to do so occasionally. Peter's whining continued intermittently for the next few months and his mother's realistic acceptance of his unhappiness and its cause characterized the entire mother-child relationship. She remarked one day, "I'm sorry, Peter. I know how you feel about the baby, but I can't send her back." Although it was doubtful that the words held much meaning for him, he responded to the tone and manner by quieting.

By March Peter was reaching for toys, picking them up and banging them together. Imitative behavior was minimal, but occasionally Peter followed the teacher during the song, "hit, hit, hit the table." He repeated the motions several times and seemed delighted. When the physical therapist placed him on his hands and knees, he remained briefly in that position unassisted and reached for a toy. He was becoming more aware of his ability to interact with materials. He threw a wheel shaped toy and watched it as it rolled away. He smiled with glee when the teacher rolled it back to him and his eyes followed it as he turned to watch it glide by them. By the middle of April he was less involved in throwing objects, and spent short periods of time placing pans into the toy stove, removing, and replacing them.

The physical therapist continued positioning Peter on his hands and knees several times each session, and he was able to remain in that position unassisted for gradually lengthening periods of time. His legs were exhibiting more strength and muscle tone.

In playing with the blocks and the mailbox into which they fit, Peter removed the blocks from the drawer and then replaced them. When the teacher demonstrated that the blocks fit into the slots, Peter tried to remove the block by pushing his finger into the slot. She then showed him that the blocks had dropped to the drawer. When she directed his hand holding the block to the appropriate slot, Peter quickly opened the drawer to retrieve the block.

The Teacher's Daily Record reports on May 24: *Peter pulled himself along the floor more than five feet, a most exciting feat for Peter and the staff!* Within a month reports of his movement across the room to the rice mixture, to an enticing pull toy or to the snack table were routine. Imitative behavior was emerging, and he clapped his hands in response to the teacher's clapping. In May, his awareness of peers increased and he engaged in a tug-of-war with Keith over a pail of sand, raced Beth across the floor to reach the blocks, and permitted Gerald to place cylinders in the mailbox for him. He learned to reach for and then tug at the string of a pull toy to bring the toy toward him.

Figure 13-2 shows the comparative results of evaluations administered in January, July and December. When classes resumed in September, after a four week vacation, Peter immediately recognized the teacher and the therapist. The teaching and therapy strategies employed within the next three months continued to be similar to those noted earlier. Peter's progress was slow and the daily record reveals no sudden spurts in any of the evaluated areas of development.

By December, the physical therapist reported that his motor functioning had improved considerably during the year. He was creeping on his stomach to all areas of the room to seek out favorite toys and activities, but although mobility had quickened, movement still required great effort. His sitting balance and posture were also improved, and he could now pivot while sitting but could not sit up or lie down unaided. Protective responses were present but were not sufficient to prevent a fall.

When weight bearing was facilitated, Peter could stand at the table and manipulate materials; when placed on his hands and knees, he could maintain the position briefly. An increase in tone in the muscles of the lower extremities was evident.

Although Peter still continued to function within the range of profound retardation, his attention span had increased as had his awareness of his environment.

Parents

Peter's mother was a friendly affable woman who carried a great responsibility in a household of five young children yet managed to attend the HEED program with regularity. During her last pregnancy she had mentioned flippantly her attendant health problems and discomfort but rarely missed a session. After the infant's birth she juggled the baby, Peter, and the infant equipment from the car to the building and back again with the aid of her four-year-old daughter. Although she accepted graciously the help proffered by staff members and other mothers, she exuded a confidence in her own ability to manage. Her desire to provide Peter with an opportunity for

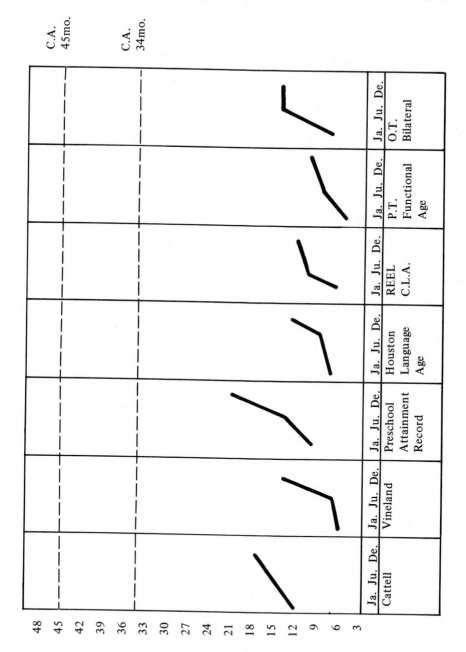

optimal development took precedence over her own comfort and convenience.

She was an active participant in the parents' group sessions which focused on feelings. She spoke of the pain she had suffered earlier when she had attempted to shield her husband and her mother from the tragedy. Her own need for empathy and support had gone unmet because of the demands upon her as wife, mother and daughter. She was a devoutly religious woman who derived comfort from her convictions, and although the many demands upon her as wife and mother sometimes created conflict with her own needs, her basic zest for life served her well in stressful situations.

Peter's parents have a satisfying marriage, and the father was often able to rearrange his schedule to provide assistance in the home so that Peter and his mother could attend class sessions without either the baby or the four-year-old sister. During the HEED experience the parents, who had intellectually perceived Peter's retardation, came to grips with the problem and seemed more reconciled to the limited prognosis. Although the child is a source of pleasure to the family, his mother was able to express realistic concerns for the future and to mention tentatively that there might be a need for temporary institutionalization at some future date.

Despite her forthright approach, Peter's mother was defended by a denial which took the form of a flippant anecdotal recounting of unpleasant or unhappy experiences, and her facile use of words enabled her to cover deep feelings. However, her genuine warmth and love for Peter and her frank admission of her own lapses endeared her to the staff. There was no doubt that this mother's life was filled with the responsibilities of caring for a busy active household and she freely admitted that the demands on her time at home often prevented her from carrying through on recommended developmental activities. Throughout the year her relationship with all the members of the team was cooperative and congenial and she became an effective spokesman in the community on the merits of programs such as HEED and on the need for additional community commitment to the education of young retarded children.

Peter is presently enrolled in a class for retarded children and he returns to the agency periodically for physical therapy treatments. The therapist reports that he can now support himself on his knees and play at a low table. Recently, he has learned to stand erect and maintain his balance while manipulating materials placed on the table. The therapist feels that the mother is providing Peter with good follow-through programming in the home.

TERESA: A CASE STUDY

Teresa was born after a thirty-two week gestation to an unmarried seventeen-year-old mother. The infant, who weighed two pounds and two ounces, suffered respiratory distress and remained in an incubator for two months. She received regular medical follow-up at a hospital clinic for premature babies, and although she was slow in learning to sit, her overall development was considered satisfactory.

The mother reported that she was unaware of any developmental problems until she realized that Teresa's walking was delayed. At age two-and-a-half, Teresa could crawl and walk on her knees but she had difficulty standing erect even with support because she could not place weight on her left leg. A referral to a cerebral palsy clinic was made at that time, and the evaluation revealed a diagnosis of cerebral palsy with mild paraparesis. Motor function in the arms seemed normal, hearing and vision were intact and speech was emerging. There was no drooling and no seizure activity.

The child was then referred to the Society for Crippled Children for intensive physical therapy and training in activities of daily living. The father, who attends school out of town and maintains sporadic contact with the child, was present for the in-take interview. Both he and the mother were confused about how physical therapy would help Teresa, and the father, particularly, seemed unable to grasp the explanation of the child's diagnosis. After a lengthy discussion of cerebral palsy and its symptoms as they related to Teresa, the father still appeared uncertain, and the caseworker suggested he contact the physician. Whether he followed through on this suggestion is unknown.

HEED Participation

Teresa entered HEED in May, 1973 when she was two years and nine months of age. She was a petite child, immaculately groomed, and although she clung to her mother, she was obviously alert to the new environment and eager to explore it. She crawled freely about the room and engaged herself in numerous activities but insisted that her mother remain at her side. She understood the teacher's questions and replied in a soft tone. Her mother was gentle and loving but firm in her demands. The mother's expectations occasionally seemed unrealistic to the teacher and therapist in view of Teresa's age, but the mother's deep affection for the child permeated their entire relationship.

The following are the results of Teresa's initial evaluations:

Cattell Infant Intelligence Scale	30 months
Vineland Social Maturity Scale	24 months
Preschool Attainment Record	27 months
Physical Therapy	14.5 months
Occupational Therapy	27 months
Houston Test for Language Development	20 months
Bzoch-League Receptive-Expressive Emergent Language Scale	33 months

Figure 13-3 shows the comparative results of evaluation administered in April and December.

During the first few weeks Teresa continued to cling to her mother and to exclude everyone else, staff and peers. At first, the mother seemed to enjoy Teresa's dependence, but after the first few weeks she appeared determined to be cooperative, and she often persuaded the child to take part in an activity with a staff person. For example, Teresa refused the teacher's invitation to paint, but at her mother's insistence she acquiesced reluctantly. When the mother was reassured that Teresa did

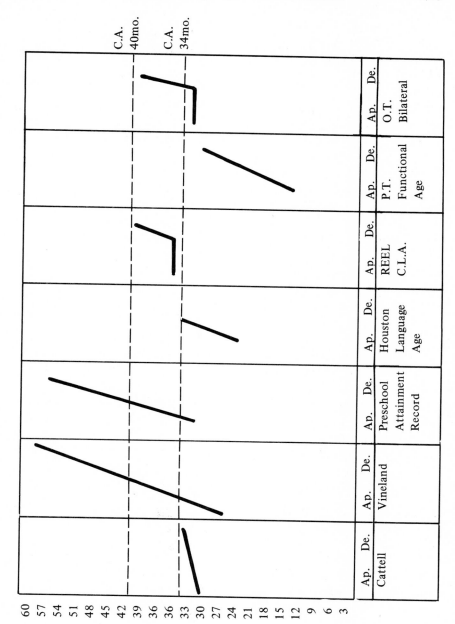

have the option of making a decision, the mother listened politely but continued directing the child to comply.

Initially, Teresa's mother had reacted toward the other mothers with diffidence, and because of Teresa's need for her in the classroom, she had had no real opportunity, nor had she evidenced any desire, to talk with them. Two weeks after the entry date, with staff encouragement, she left the room to have coffee with the other mothers. Teresa screamed and could not be comforted until her mother returned, but after the mother's return, both Teresa and her mother were more relaxed than either had ever been before. From that time Teresa was willing to interact with the teacher and the therapist for short periods of time, always returning to her mother. Gradually, her mother was able to leave the room for longer intervals. She often retired to the observation room where she maintained a keen interest in her daughter's activities. It seemed to the staff that Teresa's mother was subordinating the pleasure she derived from being with the child and having the child dependent upon her to her ultimate goal of encouraging Teresa to be independent.

By mid-spring Teresa enjoyed trying all suggested activities and was especially delighted with those which took place out-of-doors. Although her affect was usually flat, she became actively involved in all aspects of the daily routine. She enjoyed working with puzzles, creating with paint and soap suds, participating in gross motor activities such as climbing up the slide and crawling through the tunnel. She maintained a slightly suspicious attitude toward the teacher, perhaps a resentment at being separated from her mother, but this in no way impeded Teresa's continued involvement with all the available materials.

Her verbal exhanges with staff and peers expanded, and she spontaneously communicated in two and three word phrases which could be clearly understood although she still spoke softly. Her initial reaction to classmates had been withdrawal, and she remained somewhat distrustful of them, but by July she tolerated their approaching her and joining in parallel play. She asserted ownership of a toy she was holding when it was coveted by another child and even demonstrated aggressive behavior to a classmate whose toy she wanted. Teresa's mother refused to permit the child to snatch toys from other children, and at one point slapped Teresa when she caused another child distress.

Parents

Teresa and her mother had lived with the maternal grandmother and her young children. The grandmother's lack of control over her children and the ensuing chaos within the household frustrated Teresa's mother who feared ill effects for her own child. When with casework support she recognized her inability to improve conditions for her mother and her siblings, she secured an apartment for herself and her child. Despite her fear of the neighborhood and her loneliness, she was pleased with her clean attractive apartment because it afforded her the independence she needed to assume direction of her own and her child's lives.

Both Teresa and her mother were shy when they first entered the HEED program; the mother was inclined at first to shield her child and seemed to enjoy the fact that Teresa preferred her to any staff member. However, as the mother relaxed in the setting, she gained confidence in the staff and then responded with eagerness to their suggestions for expanding the HEED experiences into the home. The teacher demonstrated ways Teresa could help in dressing and undressing herself, and the mother began to utilize them. She also learned from the teacher simple games for teaching the matching of colors, and she played them with Teresa at home. Although she had been encouraging her child to walk, she accepted the therapist's recommendation to stress knee walking first to help Teresa gain strength and balance. In the course of the HEED experience, this mother's attitude of aloofness changed to genuine cordiality.

She became a careful observer of teaching and therapy techniques and by the end of the year worked effectively as an assisting adult within the classroom. The staff noted that her manner of managing an altercation between two children was similar to their own. She began to use distraction in favor of confrontation and punishment when a dispute arose, and the teacher and therapist observed that her conversations with the children were modeled after theirs. She expressed a desire to work with young children in a nursery school, and the staff encouraged her to investigate the possibility for such a career.

In January, 1974 Teresa entered the agency nursery school. Because she had visited the class many times during the previous two months, she was familiar with the teachers and children and the setting. Her mother accompanied her for the first few sessions after which Teresa was content to come on the school bus unattended by her mother. Her teachers report that she is an interested observer in the classroom. She participates eagerly in all teacher directed activities but has not yet begun to initiate activities. Although she is not demanding of adult attention, her active involvement in a project or a task is dependent upon teacher direction or suggestion.

Although interaction with peers is limited, Teresa does not seem threatened by her classmates or by the exuberant boisterous activities in which they sometimes engage. However, she waits for the teachers' suggestion before she approaches a group of children who are involved in interactive play. Her teachers feel that this is a manifestation of shyness and may also reflect her mother's expectation that before initiating an activity she wait for adult sanction. It is anticipated that as she becomes more familiar with the setting, she will participate more freely. Teresa's standing balance and assisted ambulation have improved, and she is now standing alone and taking a few rapid steps.

CHAPTER 14

EVALUATION OF PROJECT HEED: THE CHILDREN

IN THIS CHAPTER SUMMARIES of data obtained concerning measured growth of HEED children along several dimensions are presented. HEED participants are first considered as a group and statistical analyses are reported. Table I presents descriptive data concerning all those children who were enrolled in Project HEED from January through December, 1973.

In view of the heterogeneity of needs and levels of functioning presented by these children, however, it was of interest to analyze in a more detailed fashion some of these diverse patterns of gain. For this purpose, descriptive profiles of relatively homogeneous clusters of children were constructed. Three of these clusters which appeared to reflect especially distinct patterns are described.

COMPARISONS OF GAINS ANTICIPATED AND GAINS ACHIEVED

Diagnostic assessment of language development, gross motor functioning, and perceptual-motor development and activities of daily living were conducted by the speech pathologist, physical therapist, and occupational therapist, respectively. Although the results of these assessments were used primarily in a formative manner with respect to determination of progress of each child in light of his individual needs and disability, overall comparisons of pre-test and post-test performances were also made as an index of program effectiveness.

In Table II, group data are presented in the form of *Test Age* equivalent earned (that is, age equivalent score) on both the pre and post-measure. The intervening time between measures

TABLE I
Characteristics of the HEED Children: 1973

Child	Age	IQ	Entry Date	Months in HEED	Diagnosis and Presenting Prob.
1	21 mos	44	1/20	12	Cerebral palsy: spastic diplegia. Severe retardation
2	24 mos	100	9/11	3	Cerebral palsy: spastic paraplegia
3	28 mos	74	1/8	12	Cerebral palsy: spastic diplegia
4	25 mos	88	9/13	3	Cerebral palsy: spastic quadriplegia
5	24 mos	93	9/10	3	Cerebral palsy: spastic diplegia
6	38 mos	21	6/26	6	Hallerman-Streiff Syndrome
7	22 mos	59	2/13	11	Cerebral palsy: spastic quadriplegia
8	29 mos	56	10/10	2	Cerebral palsy
9	24 mos	96	9/24	3	London Flu, brain damage
10	30 mos	78	10/25	2	Cerebral palsy: spastic diplegia
11	32 mos	89	4/30	8	Hypotonia
12	32 mos	91	5/7	7	Cerebral palsy: spastic paraplegia
13*	34 mos	29	1/4	12	Mental-motor retardation
14*	48 mos	43	1/3	12	Cerebral palsy: spastic quadreplegia
15	38 mos	66	4/10	8	Congenital heart; right hemiparesis
16	22 mos	—	10/1	3	Cerebral palsy: right hemiplegia Seizures
[1]17*	35 mos	99	1/2	12	Right leg amputee
[1]18	44 mos	55	1/3	12	Spina bifida, shunted hydrocephalus
19	36 mos	71	1/22	12	Cerebral palsy: cerebellar ataxia
[1]20	49 mos	71	1/3	3	Hydrocephalus, shunted
[1]21	31 mos	80	1/8	12	Encephalopathy
[1]22	31 mos	100	1/2	7	Cerebral palsy: spastic quadriplegia

*Prior membership in original pilot project: The Developmental Group

1-Transferred to regular Nursery School and therapy services prior to December 1973

2-No longer in HEED: outpatient only, periodic

TABLE II
Expected and Observed Gains Based on
Special Therapies Diagnostic Evaluations:
t-tests of Differences Between Correlated Means

Assessment Dimension	Pre-test		Post-test		Expected Gain		Observed Gain		t-ratio
	Mean	Var.	Mean	Var.	Mean	Var.	Mean	Var.	
Physical Therapy: Functional Age	11.78	4.62	16.83	6.48	2.43	1.48	5.08	2.88	2.65**
Occupational Therapy: Unilateral Skills	16.50	8.20	22.56	8.08	4.01	2.25	6.06	3.09	2.08*
O.T.: Bilateral Skills	15.97	8.39	23.12	8.74	3.83	2.56	7.41	5.39	2.32*
O.T.: Activities of Daily Living	17.33	6.50	21.62	7.79	4.09	2.03	4.25	3.06	0.17 (NS)
Speech: Houston Language Age	14.56	7.09	20.25	8.27	3.27	1.88	5.69	4.13	2.06*

N=16, df=15
*p<.05
**p<.01

varies as a function of each child's length of time in the program. Analyses were based on a comparison of each child's *Expected Gain* and *Observed Gain* on each respective measure. Expected Gain for each child is computed by determining his TA/CA ration (age equivalent score earned at pre-test divided by chronological age at pre-test) and by multiplying this quotient by the number of months between his pre and post-measure (i.e. length of time in program). It is assumed that the child's prior rate of development in that area of function is thereby taken into account as a predictive index of how rapidly his development would proceed were there no intervention (i.e. as a function of normal maturation and experience). The Observed Gain is the gain (expressed in months) reflected in his actual performance on the post-test measure.

Although other dimensions of the physical therapy assessment are described in the section presenting analyses of small group progress, the physical therapy index of central concern is that of Functional Age. This is the score computed on the basis of activities accomplished within normal limits and average time as well as those accomplished, but awkwardly or with difficulty. Thus, this index reflects what the child has learned to accomplish within the limits imposed by his handicapping condition.

As Table II shows, the group as a whole achieved a mean gain in functional age of 5.08 months, moving from an average level of functioning of 11.78 months to 16.83 months on the post-measure. This gain occurred over an average time span of 6.88 months, and can be contrasted with the expected gain for that period which was estimated to be only 2.43 months. The difference between the expected and observed gain scores is significant ($p < .01$, df = 16, one-tailed test). All children experienced an increase, and for all but two the increase was greater than would have been anticipated without intervention through HEED. Although nearly all these children continue to function at a level substantially below their chronological age in terms of motor skills, ambulation, and balance, they appear as a group to have progressed substantially during the time they were enrolled in HEED (from two to eleven months). Nearly one half of these seventeen children gained as many months or more in their equivalent scores as they had actually been in the program, although none was expected to do so.

The progress made by the children in fine motor control and perceptual-motor coordination is reflected by the comparisons shown in Table II which also shows similar comparisons for the Activities of Daily Living dimension of the occupational therapy assessment. As these data show, substantial progress was made in terms of both unilateral and bilateral skills, but change was not significant for the ADL dimension. Further discussion of the lack of significant gains in ADL on the part of many children in the program is provided in the following pages. It may be noted that, in contrast to the other areas in which gains were sought and were in fact made by virtually all HEED participants, only about one third of the children gained more in ADL than they were expected to gain.

For Unilateral Skills, the difference between expected and observed gain means was significant ($p<.05$, df = 15, one-tailed test). Twelve of the sixteen children, or 75 percent, gained more in unilateral skill functioning than would have been predicted if there was no intervention. The average gain observed was six months during an average intervention time period of 7.63 months. The average gain predicted to occur during this period was four months. There was a wide range of variation, not only in participation time, but also in entry level and final level. One child, in the program for one year and expected, based on initial performance, to progress less than two and one-half months, progressed during this period at a normal rate. Nine of the sixteen children progressed at a rate commensurate with their actual program participation time, although their prior development had been at a substantially slower rate. In fact pre-test scores suggested that only three had developed in this area at the rate of 80 percent or more of their chronological age. More than one-third had achieved less than 50 percent of the accomplishments associated with their chronological age norms at the time of initial assessment, or before entering HEED.

Similar results were obtained for the dimension of bilateral skills. Again, 75 percent increased more than anticipated, based on entry performance level, and the difference between mean expected and observed gain was significant ($p<.05$, df $= 15$, one-tailed test).

These patterns of gain reveal significant improvement in upper extremity motor functioning, both unilateral and bilateral, which can be inferred to be associated with the intervention. More specific patterns of progress are reflected in the discussions of small homogeneous groups which follow. For each of these two areas of concern, a broad range of individual differences in needs and growth patterns was revealed. This is exemplified by the instance of one child who progressed from the point of total inability to use a paralyzed arm to compensatory bilateral functioning. The average bilateral upper extremity motor functioning of the group as a whole, based on its mean level of post-test, was commensurate with average program participation time, with nearly one-half the group progressing at an even more rapid rate.

In terms of language development, as assessed by the Houston Test for Language Development, group differences also reached significance, and it can be inferred that HEED intervention was instrumental in this area as well. Twelve of the sixteen children, or three-fourths, progressed at a more rapid rate than would have been anticipated based on their entry levels. The expected vs. observed gain mean difference was statistically significant ($p<.05$, df $= 15$, one-tailed test). In the area of language functioning, intragroup variability was again the rule, with one child gaining seventeen months (i.e. literally acquiring functional language) and three children continuing to operate at an essentially pre-lingual level after five, eight, and ten months, respectively, of program participation time. It should be noted that all but two of these sixteen children manifested serious or severe language and/or speech disability or retardation, either as a central or associated aspect of their primary handicapping condition. More detailed analyses of language-related problems and gains are provided in the discussion which follows.

The *Teacher's Periodic Checklist*, an instrument designed especially for formative assessment of needs and progress of individual children in Project HEED, was administered by the teacher to each child upon entering the program and then successively at six month intervals. Consequently, some of the children whose ratings are shown in Table I were rated twice while others had three ratings. The table compares first and last ratings, expressed as percentages of the total rating score possible in each of the four dimensions of Social Adaptation, Exploration of Environment, Self-awareness and Body Mastery, and Cognitive Skills. Assignment of items to each of the four categories was done on the basis of face validity, and there is some overlapping between categories.

Detailed discussion of the nature of items and their rationale for inclusion was provided in Chapter 4. As an evaluative procedure, the Checklist presented serious limitations in that no norms are as yet available and it is impossible to determine to what extent gains are a function of program impact, rather than normal maturation and experience outside HEED, since no control group was available. The Checklist is primarily a tool for the identification of specific needs and accomplishments of individualized programming within the group setting.

As Table III shows, however, pre and post-mean differences were significant for all four dimensions when the group is considered as a whole. It is clear that the development of nearly all HEED participants, based on the teacher's perception, progressed markedly in all areas, particularly the areas of Self-awareness and Body Mastery. These changes are striking both from the standpoint of their near universality and from that of their absolute magnitude, especially in individual instances. Individual and homogeneous group patterns are perhaps more meaningful, but this overall comparison serves to convey the teacher's impression that marked progress had taken place in the ability of most of the children to adapt to a social milieu, to explore, to be aware of self and to gain mastery over some body functions, and to develop a basic cognitive repertoire upon which subsequent conceptual attainment might build.

TABLE III
Education Assessment: Teacher's Periodic Checklist
Pre and Post Ratings for Social Adaptation,
Exploration of Environment, Self-Awareness
and Body Mastery and Cognitive Skills
(Percents of Total Possible Scores)

Child	Time In Program (mos)	Social Adaptation		Explor. of Environ.		Self-Aware. Body Mast.		Cog. Skills	
		Pre	Post	Pre	Post	Pre	Post	Pre	Post
1	11	23	12	18	15	10	33	4	1
2	3	29	58	59	72	47	73	34	42
3	3	74	82	67	77	53	97	45	48
4	8	36	69	56	56	39	57	27	45
5	8	63	84	62	56	62	97	43	70
6	8	66	80	51	84	58	83	58	78
7	11	20	79	77	67	24	90	13	63
8	11	40	73	26	64	43	93	20	56
9	11	40	92	31	97	46	100	12	73
10	11	63	100	56	97	61	100	4	98
11	11	53	75	23	46	36	53	18	40
12	11	30	17	10	5	18	27	5	6
13	11	47	70	54	38	59	77	39	34
14	6	61	66	58	59	50	67	31	57
15	3	50	56	56	67	53	60	40	49
16	1	36	79	72	90	43	97	56	69
17	2	61	79	54	74	43	93	44	64
18	7	85	89	69	92	53	100	58	94
Mean		48.72	70.00	49.94	64.22	44.33	77.61	30.61	54.83
Variance		17.78	22.35	19.12	25.19	14.24	22.75	18.06	24.87
t-ratio		t=3.07**		t=1.86*		t=5.11***		t=3.25**	

*p<.05
**p<.005
***p<.001

ANALYSES OF CHILDREN'S PROGRESS BY SMALL HOMOGENEOUS GROUPS

In this section analyses of changes reflected in the educational, physical therapy, occupational therapy, and speech pathology assessments are presented in order to illustrate individual patterns of growth. For the purpose of this analysis, the children were assigned to groups of four, five, or six, each of which reflected significant commonalities in terms of primary disability, level of general intellectual ability, and time in progress. The general characteristics of each group are discussed briefly.

Group I

Group I comprises five children who score within the normal range of intellectual functioning according to the Cattell Infant Scale. Their IQ's on entry ranged from 89 to 100. Given their motor handicaps and consequent experiential limitations, their scores are probably depressed estimates of their intellectual capacity.

The individual medical diagnoses are spastic diplegia, spastic paraplegia, spastic quadriplegia, hypotonia and a right leg amputation resulting from cardiovascular disease. Their primary disability essentially involves their motor functioning, with less pronounced effects upon sensory systems. The most obvious distinction between these children and non-handicapped children is that they sit, crawl and walk later. All children in Group I have leg involvement and some limited hand involvement. The extent to which their functional disability is defined by limited and delayed walking is suggested by a comparison of their physical therapy and occupational therapy scores and their chronological ages at entry. At entry, the mean chronological age for this group was 31.4 months. The mean physical equivalent age was 10.56 months while the mean occupational therapy scores for bilateral and unilateral manipulation were each 21.6 months. The physical therapy measure shows the group functioning 20.84 months below its chronological age. In contrast, the occupational therapy measure shows the group functioning 9.8 months below its chronological age.

In general, the sensory systems of the group members do not seem affected by their primary handicapping condition. One child did suffer from extremely poor vision and had problems with eye-hand coordination. Another child had a history of eye surgery, but her behavior in the HEED setting did not suggest a visual problem which would interfere with her functioning in the classroom. No child gave an indication of a hearing loss, and only one child seemed to have an expressive disorder, and his progress on the Houston suggests it is amenable to therapy.

This is a group of children whose physical impairment is limited to their ability to get around independently. However, their handicap did not greatly limit their ability to interact with their environment in order to make the sensory and manipulative discriminations necessary for learning.

Physical Therapy

The Physical Therapy measure yields four age scores: a basal, or level at which all items are passed, the level of highest achievement, or level of the most advanced physical action, the equivalent age or age level at which the handicapped child does things in a normal manner, and the functional age, or level at which the child masters a task, in any manner. At entry, the mean basal age was 12 months and the mean level of highest accomplishment (L.H.A.) was 19.8 months. At the final testing, the mean basal had risen 2.4 months to 14.4 months while the mean L.H.A. had risen 16.2 months to 36 months. The mean range of the group's activity had been stretched 13.8 months. Within that range the mean equivalent age rose 5.04 months, twice the mean expected gain of 2.47 months.

Similarly, the mean functional age rose 6.08 months, almost twice the mean expected gain of 3.59 months. The relatively parallel rise of equivalent and functional ages suggests that these intellectually normal children used their physical capacity comparatively (probably fully) at entry and throughout the program. The doubling of their rate of progress is assumed to reflect the effectiveness of the therapy and the HEED environment.

Occupational Therapy

The occupational therapy measure yields scores for a level of physical readiness, levels of unilateral and bilateral manipulatory scores and a score for activities of daily living. The group mean gain in unilateral activities was approximated the expected gain. The group mean gain for bilateral activities was 6.25 months or 1.36 months more than the expected gain. The greater gain in bilateral activities might reflect the influence of the HEED environment which encouraged purposeful exploration of toys and which included creative activities which involved both hands.

The mean gain in Activities of Daily Living was less than the expected gain. In only one case did a child achieve more than his expected gain, and that child was temperamentally vigorous and self-directing. With the exception of that child, all children's manipulatory scores are closer to their chronological age than their A.D.L. scores. Several factors may contribute to the lag in A.D.L. The HEED curriculum with its plethora of manipulatory toys and emphasis on physical therapy reinforced the occupational therapy which was directed to bilateral manipulation more than it reinforced A.D.L. Many of the mothers in this group, despite encouragement, had difficulty in stressing self-care, and one seemed to discourage it. Hence A.D.L. activities which depended upon home follow-up lagged.

Language

Two language measures were administered. One, the Bzoch-League Receptive-Expressive Emergent Language Scale (REEL), is a parent report scale, and the other, the Houston, is an objective test administered directly to the child. The REEL yields three age level scores, one reflecting receptive language, one expressive language and a combined language age score which averages the others. On all three measures the children's final scores closely reflected their chronological age at the initial testing. On the CLA, the parents of three children initially estimated them to be five, eight and two months below their chronological age in language functioning, while two rated scores above their chronological age. At final testing, however, no child was rated above his chronological age.

The relative decline in language may reflect the parents' acceptance of their children's language. This interpretation is substantiated by the general convergence of the final REEL combined language age and Houston language age scores. On the REEL combined language age, the final scores range from 36 to 25.5 months, while on the Houston they range from 33 to 21 months.

The Houston scores are slightly lower than the REEL, which may reflect the tendency of children this age to withhold speech in an unfamiliar situation. The Houston mean basal age score rose strikingly while the upper scores remained generally constant. The exception to the trend was a two-year-old child functioning at an age level of one. In keeping with the expansive pattern of language during the second and third years, her upper score rose to six months in four months while her basal remained constant. It is interesting to note that this child's language range widened while the near three to four-year-old's language range narrowed. This suggests a trend of language development, a period of rapidly expanding and relatively erratic use of language forms which become more integrated as the child nears age four. The pattern suggests a perhaps delayed but basically normal language usage as characteristic of this group. The closeness of the observed gain and the expected gain reinforces the picture of this group as basically normal in the language area.

The Teacher's Periodic Checklist

All individuals gained in all areas assessed via the Teacher's Periodic Checklist. The mean gain in percent of total possible score in self-awareness and body mastery was 19.55 percent; in exploration of the environment it was 22.14 percent; in social adaptation the mean gain was 38.42 percent, and in cognitive skills the gain averaged 32.08 percent. When this group entered HEED, its highest mean percent of the total possible score was in self-awareness; at final testing the highest mean percent was found in social adaptation. The change may reflect the socializing experience of the HEED environment and a normal developmental trend of lessening egocentrism.

Group II

IQ scores on entry cluster around the 70's. The exception, a severely involved quadriplegic, initially tested at 43 on the Cattell, but later achieved a Peabody Picture Vocabulary Test IQ of 69. Since the Cattell makes more motor demands than the Peabody, it seems reasonable to infer that the Cattell score reflects her physical limitation.

Primary medical diagnoses are of cerebral palsy with spastic diplegia and spastic quadriplegia, congenital heart defect and right hemiparesis, encephalopathy, cerebellar ataxia, and shunted hydrocephalus. All children suffered motor limitations. Three had marked hand involvement which limited their ability to manipulate objects. The group's primary diagnoses leave room to suspect generalized damage to the central nervous system. Aside from the obvious limitations and distortions of sensory feedback imposed by conditions such as hemiparesis and ataxia, some of the children had histories of seizures, and others had periods of blanking that led the staff to suspect possible seizure activity. Their medical conditions imply that these children may have difficulty in organizing environmental stimuli and responding to it.

Physical Therapy

On entry, the mean basal age was nine months and the level of highest accomplishment was 17.5. Several children had identical scores reflecting the general evenness of the group range. The final basal and level of highest achievement scores reflect the same general evenness; the range of activity is widened to 10.5 months, and the whole shows improvement. The final mean basal is 13.5 months and the final L.H.A. is 24 months. Four members of the group gained from 2.8 to 3.6 times their expected gain on the L.H.A. while two members did not achieve theirs.

Of the children who did not achieve the predicted gain, one was a shunted hydrocephalic, and the other a severely involved quadriplegic. The handicaps of these two group members may have set ceilings on their achievement. The presence of a ceiling to normal physical development is seen in the lack of progress on the equivalent age. Only two children achieved more than their expected gain and the rest achieved less. The mean observed gain of 2.02 months was only 60 percent of a meager expected gain of 3.37 months for a twelve month period. However, every child achieved more than his expected gain in functional age, and some achieved many times their expected gain.

The spread of final scores is greater than their initial spread, which may reflect the individual group members' differing abilities to profit from the therapy and the HEED environment. While their equivalent age remained relatively static, therapy may have enabled them to extend their functional performance levels according to their individual capacities. However, the determining nature of their physical handicap remains evident in the basically consistent orderings and in the distance between individual's functional and equivalent age scores. The child who scored lowest on her functional age scored lowest on her equivalent age, and her functional age is closest to her equivalent age.

Occupational Therapy

With the consistent exceptions of two children on the measure for bilateral manipulation, a marked and steady increment was found between the second and third testing. The pattern may reflect the impact of therapy and the HEED environment on children who had been functioning well below their capacity. On the measure for bilateral manipulation the two children who show the greatest initial gains are the two most physically handicapped in terms of bilateral manipulation. One suffered hemiparesis and the other severe spasticity. Both children needed a good deal of encouragement before they would engage in bimanual activities. The spastic child was very passive, and the hemiplegic tended to reject his involved side, characteristically holding his involved arm behind him.

In all areas the group achieved better than the mean expected gain. The mean expected gain for unilateral manipulation was 5.43 months, and the mean observed gain was 7.45 months. The mean expected gain for bilateral manipulation was 4.94 months, and the mean observed gain was 10.71 months. For Activities of Daily Living the mean expected gain was 5.23, and the mean observed gain was 6.09 months. With the exception of bilateral activities, the means tend to be misleading because some children achieved a great deal more than the expected gain, while others failed to achieve it. In general, children with severe physical and motivational handicaps made the greatest gains, while those children who were more able made less gains.

Language

All members of this group have a history of irregular language development. On intake, most of the mothers reported acquisition and then loss of simple nouns such as *dog, allow, drink* and phrases such as *I want a*. Only a child who lost language after suffering a cardiovascular accident had a medical history which supplied a clear cause for the language loss. However, many of the children were suspected of having mild seizures. As they progressed through the year, two children showed unusual amounts of echoing, and one tended to refer to non-present objects and events as present. The child who suffered the CVA became dependent upon the expletive "shut-up" as an all purpose word. As a group, these children show irregular acquisition and use of language.

It is interesting to note that the parent report scales predict the language progress of this group more accurately than the objective measure administered directly to the children. The REEL receptive language age mean expected gain was 6.1 months and the children achieved a 7.5 month gain. The mean expected gain for the expressive language age was 7.4 months while the mean observed gain was 9 months. The mean expected gain for the Houston language age was 3.93 months and the observed gain was nine months. The mother's reports do not portray a large gap between receptive and expressive language. It may be that mothers were able to understand language that was relatively unintelligible, and that the therapy and the HEED environment helped to render it intelligible. There is also the probability that these children, with good reason to be unsure of their language, withheld during the initial testing. The classroom observation supports an impression of irregular but expanding language. Frequently, a parent would report the use of a noun or a verbal identification of a color before that behavior appeared in the HEED setting.

On initial testing all children scored between twenty-four and thirty-six months on the Houston upper age dimension and all were below six months on the basal. On the final testing the children grouped at thirty-six and thirty months on the upper score. Two children retained basals of below six months, two achieved basals of twelve months, and two achieved basals of eighteen months. Throughout the year, each individual's language age score rose relatively consistently. These children belatedly and awkwardly created child language from infant language.

Teacher's Periodic Checklist

The generally large gains reflected in the ratings of all but one child suggest that engagement in all four areas characterized the participation of this group. Exceptions, such as the one child in particular whose final ratings were lower in all areas, may reflect the teacher's sense that her initial judgments had been overly favorable. Only two maintained substantial gains in Exploration of Environment, perhaps reflecting some combination of actual impairment in motor exploration, motivational passivity, and/or a relatively higher degree of distractibility than is found for Group I.

Although Cognitive Skill gains during the first six months were substantial, the last rating reveals some leveling off. It is reasonable to suppose that general intellectual limitations are at least to some degree responsible for this effect. Overall, Social Adaptation reveals the greatest gain, although for two of the children a decline was perceived at mid-year, with final ratings for these children being not impressively higher than when they entered.

All six were seen to progress markedly in Self-awareness and Body Mastery, with two leveling from mid-year to the final assessment. Clinical observations of various staff members suggested an awareness of heightened motivation and involvement on the part of children in this group as they progressed in the program, suggesting a general responsiveness to most aspects of the HEED milieu. All five of these children have now entered the agency's regular nursery school program, the decision in each case having been based upon both the age of the child and a judgment that each was ready to move beyond HEED. The current functioning of at least two suggests the need for a continuation of the individualization of attention that was possible in HEED in order to effect this transition optimally.

Group III

This group consists of four severely retarded children. Their Cattell IQ's on entry ranged from 21 to 44. Their medical diagnoses are cerebral palsy with severe retardation, Hallerman-Streiff Syndrome, spastic diplegia with suspected microcephaly, and "mental motor retardation." Their primary handicap is essentially the severity of their general retardation. Compared to the children of Group I and Group II, these children have relatively able bodies which their retardation prevents them from using as a tool. All of the children maintain limited eye contact, and two of the children show symptoms of severe sensory impairment. These two exhibit marked tactile-defensiveness and inappropriate affect. To a degree, all of the children seem to reject external stimulation. Their sensory life arises from within and manifests itself in oral stimulation, masturbation, and inappropriate laughing and crying.

Physical Therapy

Despite the severity of their retardation, all children made gains in equivalent and functional ages. The mean gain in equivalent age was 2.75 months, and the mean gain in functional age was 3.5 months. On the final testing three of the children's equivalent and functional age scores are within four months of each other, and far below their chronological age. Children aged forty-six, forty-four, and thirty-two months achieved functional age scores of eight, 8.5 and 7.5 months respectively. The 3.5 month rise in the functional age score is 55 percent better than the expected gain of 1.94 months, and the 2.75 month rise in equivalent age is 45 percent better than the expected gain of 1.26 months. All children in this group appeared to benefit from physical therapy.

Occupational Therapy

The mean scores on the occupational therapy manipulatory measure are misleading, since one child made a large gain while the other children made no gains. The child who gained went from ten to eighteen months in unilateral and bilateral skills. He owed his gain to the ability to build a three block tower and to use both hands when imitating in pulling clay apart. The others' lack of growth in manipulatory skill reflects more their tendency not to act on their environment rather than a physical disability. On the Activities of Daily Living measure, the group progress is summarized in a mean gain of .5 months, well below the expected gain of 2.83 months. Many of the children have feeding problems in addition to a lack of manipulatory skills.

Language

On the REEL combined language age, the mean observed gain was 1.5 months, a little more than half a month below the expected gain of 2.14 months. The two children who lost ground on the CLA were those who show signs of severe sensory impairment. The other children gained two months more than their individual expected gains. The loss in the REEL score may show parental acceptance of the non-referent nature of their children's babbling. One mother who initially reported that her child said "da-da" reported on final testing that the child perseverated in the response after someone in-itiated it. The Houston language age shows gains on the part of all individuals with a mean gain of two months, a half month better than the expected gain. Their language remains at the babbling level. Some show interest in sounds, while others clearly babble as a manifestation of non-directed internal stimu-lation.

Teacher's Periodic Checklist

The mean percentage of the total possible score declined in all areas, excepting socialization. The Checklist, which is con-structed on the assumption that learning is the result of interac-tion with the environment, may not be suitable for severely retarded children such as these, who interact with the envi-ronment in a very limited way.

It is clinically observed that the attention of these children is primarily centered on somatic-originated stimulation, rather than external stimulation from the environment. The term *tactile-defensive* has been used to characterize the rejection of external stimulation which children such as these frequently manifest (Ayers, 1972). It is felt that the severe sensory disorders experienced by two children in this group militate against sensory transactions with the environment. At least their level of readiness to engage actively in environmental encounters and to order experiences obtained through these encounters may be such that very different program expectations and strategies, as well as measurement instruments, are called for.

The program variation initiated in response to this conclusion is described briefly in Chapter 15. It appeared clear to the staff that a scaled-down, modified nursery school program was inappropriate for children as severely impaired as these, and that a sensory approach, with reduced general stimulation, would more nearly meet their needs.

The three groups described in the preceding pages appear to manifest distinctive characteristics which may suggest the need for distinctly different ameliorative approaches. This is particularly apparent in the case of the third group whose profile is presented. In the course of the first project year, a gradual shift in emphasis for children with these characteristics evolved, a shift which became articulated and formally incorporated in the program design near the end of the year. The resultant changes in focus and in logistics are discussed in the concluding chapter.

The final chapter also summarizes and interprets evaluative data presented here in relationship to the program objectives originally formulated. In this regard, program impact is assessed also in terms of its perceived effects on those parents who participated. Although both in theory and in practice the project staff conceived the parent and child components as inseparable and interdependent, distinct objectives were formulated and evaluation procedures implemented in order to gauge the impact of HEED on parents, as well as their children.

Using the participating parents as a major data source, two distinct procedures were carried out. First, it was particularly essential to ascertain how these parents saw the program and their own role in it. An anonymous questionnaire was used in order to elicit candid responses to open-ended and forced choice questions concerning various aspects of the program. Secondly, the HEED caseworker was asked to assess current needs and areas of progress or growth for each individual parent participating in the program. The necessary subjectivity of both procedures, the former utilizing a self-report format, the latter seeking to employ the clinical sensitivity and acumen of the professional most closely involved with these parents, unquestionably mitigates the validity of conclusions drawn based on these data. However, these procedures proved extremely useful both in the formative processes of individual goal-setting and program review, and also summatively in ascertaining what had been accomplished in the program during its first year.

Finally, conclusions drawn and recommendations offered based on the HEED evaluative study are related to the several themes delineated throughout the book relating to intervention which is designed to influence the physical and psychological development of young children with handicaps. As has been suggested, many of these themes are applicable to diverse efforts in early childhood and special education and to interdisciplinary team functioning in general.

CHAPTER 15

CONCLUSIONS: THE IMPACT OF COMPREHENSIVE INTERVENTION

PERHAPS THE MOST SIGNIFICANT aspect to staff of their experiences in Project HEED during its first year was the conscientious, perhaps dedicated, involvement of most of the participating parents as partners in the intervention process. There is no doubt that these parents left their own mark on the operation of the program and contributed greatly to the professionals' ability to carry out their work with children. This involvement is illustrated by one mother who, on her own initiative, developed and edited a parents' newsletter which was published periodically. This mother, and others who worked with her on this project, contributed greatly to the personalized and humanistic tone of the project by, for example, printing occasional special features on various staff members and personal notes concerning activities of both parents and staff.

In terms of more objective evidence of parent cooperation and involvement, the consistency of attendance of most parents may be cited. Table IV presents a summary of the attendance record of each child enrolled in HEED during the year.

Anticipated problems with regular attendance due to the children's young age, transportation problems, multiple medical problems and susceptibility to upper respiratory ailments, the necessity for parent attendance, and a variety of additional factors would presumably make attendance difficult, especially during the winter months. Although, given these considerations, the record of consistency of attendance was considered unusually good, the spurious effects of high necessary absenteeism on the part of a very small number tend to mask the extraordinary consistency of participation of the group as a whole.

TABLE IV
Attendance of All HEED Participants*

Child	Possible Sessions	Sessions Attended	Percent of Attendance
1	75	61	81.3
2	27	27	100
3	74	70	94.5
4	21	21	100
5	27	22	81.4
6	30	28	93.3
7	65	31	40.7
8	18	15	82.2
9	23	19	82.5
10	14	12	85.7
11	55	32	58.1
12	53	40	75.4
13	77	66	85.7
14	77	71	92.1
15	50	43	86
16	21	9	42.8
17	26	13	50
18	47	24	51
19	42	35	83.3
20	47	29	61.7
21	46	42	91.3
22	48	41	87.6
Mean	43.77	34.14	78%

*January 1, 1973 to December 31, 1973

Table IV also serves to show precisely how many actual sessions comprised the treatment program for each child. Over the course of the entire year, the range of possible sessions was from eighteen to seventy-seven, with a range of from as few as nine to as many as seventy-one attended. Using the August "break" as a natural transitional time, several HEED children were moved into the regular nursery school and special therapy programs at this time, creating openings for other children.

ASSESSING THE IMPACT OF HEED ON PARENTS

Through the casework process, areas of need and of progress of HEED parents, as perceived from the caseworker's perspective, were assessed. The scale employed for this purpose was devised specifically for use in the project primarily in order to provide a useful clinical tool for the caseworker in charting the course to be followed with each parent.

This assessment device continues to be subjected to crucial areas, to suggest an inaccurate picture, or to be otherwise inadequate. Since its primary utility is as an individual, clinical technique, the scale was difficult to use for purposes of assessing group phenomena. Although various subcategorical ratings were provided, therefore, these were compressed into more general ratings. Inclusion within the rating category *Still major concern/little progress* suggests that the item may represent either a major problem or an area in which improvement is needed, but the individual's present functioning is not adequate and/or reveals little progress. The second rating category, *Fluctuations/some progress*, denotes inconsistent functioning but that progress has been made. *Progress/adequate* denotes that an individual's functioning is *both* adequate and manifests growth.

The Casework Assessment ratings are summarized in terms of five primary dimensions. For each of these dimensions, rating scores for all parents (N = 21) and for those parents who had been in the program more than six months (N = 10) were considered separately. Parents in the 6 mos. + group had been previously rated in July, 1973; thus their ratings reflect a comparative judgment based upon the prior rating.

Dimension 1: The Acceptance-Denial Continuum

Progress made by those in the program more than six months, and thus rated for the second time, was believed to have occurred in terms of their ability to recognize their child's handicap and the limits imposed thereby on his potential accomplishments. However, even some of these parents still found it difficult to think in terms of realistic future planning, and the caseworker believed that a degree of denial was manifest in the inability of at least two parents to share recollections of their early experiences upon learning of the child's problem. The extent to which many of the parents, one third to one half of the total group, were able to cope effectively with reactions of strangers and of relatives concerning the child continued to be a source of uncertainty for the caseworker.

Dimension 2: Expression of Feelings

It is probable that feelings of ambivalence pervade all close relationships, but certainly those between parents and children. When the child has a serious physical problem, such conflicts are greatly exacerbated. Based upon the assumption that it is desirable to be able to express feelings of guilt, anxiety, anger, and frustration concerning one's child and the parenting role, the caseworker felt that about one half of the group had not as yet been able to vent these feelings adequately. Greatest progress seemed to have been made in parents' ability to discuss individual and specific child management and child rearing problems and their experiences with hospitalization, surgery, bracing and similar events.

Many were also felt to have revealed insight in the form of a recognition of their own past and current feelings of frustration and depression, although progress here, and generally in expression of affect, was considered to be irregular and marked by fluctuations in more than one half of the parents. Five parents (one fourth of the group) revealed apparent difficulty in discussing with their spouse the child's problems, although this continued to be a problem for only two who were in the program more than six months.

Dimension 3: Functioning with a Handicapped Child

Inter-parental communication concerning the handling of the child also emerged as a problem in terms of this broad dimension. For nearly one-half the group, it was an area of great need and little progress, or else was unknown to the caseworker. Father interest *per se* was, in about one-half the cases, an area of apparent fluctuation and/or moderate progress. Putting into practice the advice for home management gained through HEED or other professional sources was apparently being accomplished to at least some degree, but with a few exceptions.

The HEED messages concerning the need for appropriate environmental stimulation were believed translated into parental efforts at home in more than one-half the cases to a high degree, however, and to some degree by most. Growth in terms of positive orientation toward the child's psychological well-being and recognition of his individuality was also reflected in various other ways, including awareness of his likes and dislikes and appropriate handling in light of awareness of child developmental needs.

Most appeared to be functioning well, in addition, with respect to their expressed recognition of the positive aspects of their parenting role, their expression of acceptance of the child rather than rejection, their ability to effect separation from the child, and their ability to apply appropriate limits in managing his behavior. For many, especially those relatively new to the program, the need to provide adequate peer contact for their child appeared to require attention, although this need could be met, at least in part, through the program itself.

Child care areas of nutrition, sleep, and cleanliness were being handled adequately and/or apparent progress was being made by seventy-five percent or more of the total group, although each of these continued to be a problem for one or two. Eight of the ten parents in HEED for more than six months, and more than one-half the total group, appeared to be functioning well in terms of providing for the special needs of a handicapped child with ingenuity and imagination.

Dimension 4: Functioning in Regard to Personal Relationships

That many of the parents were deriving personal benefits from their associations gained through HEED was suggested in various ways. Meaningful and/or constructive participation in parent group meetings, informal associations with HEED staff appeared to be a source of satisfaction or growth for virtually all, especially those in the program six months or longer. Relationships with other parents and with staff members appeared to represent the most positive areas. Progress in or adequacy of relationships outside HEED was believed somewhat more tenuous, and it was not known in twelve instances whether a meaningful friendship existed.

Dimension 5: Functioning in Other Aspects of Living

A degree of uncertainty concerning the lives of HEED parents in other areas of living was also revealed in that it was not known whether one-half the total group were making effective use of community resources, such as the church or recreational facilities, in seeking personal fulfillment and satisfaction outside their parenting role.

It was felt that most (two thirds of the total and eight of the ten in HEED six months or longer) were, in general, now coping reasonably effectively with their personal situation, with several functioning quite well. However, for several, serious difficulties in personal functioning indirectly related to the role of parent of a handicapped child persisted, including marital problems and difficulty in the handling of other children in the family.

Some further interpretation of these general findings obtained via the caseworker's assessment is provided with reference to those objectives originally formulated for the parent component of Project HEED and considered as evaluative criteria. This source of data, despite its limitations and its primarily clinical function, has served to provide some indications of the degree of success of the project in attaining its objectives for parents of young handicapped children. The implications of these data contribute toward the general assessment of program effectiveness, together with a variety of objective and impressionistic indicators.

THE PROGRAM AS VIEWED BY THE PARENTS

In addition to the importance attached by the staff to their own observations of positive changes observed in the children, the perceptions of parents were of primary interest for two basic reasons. First, it was felt that parents were in the best position to identify growth and change in their own child and to interpret the ways in which the Project HEED might be contributing to such change and growth. Secondly, since HEED was geared to the needs of the parents themselves, as well as those of their children, the views of parents were essential in determining to what extent and in what ways the project might be serving them.

Project staff were also desirous of obtaining feedback which might influence the continuing process of redefining and reshaping the approach. Therefore, in a real sense parental feedback was considered an essential facet of a meaningful program, particularly a program which was intended to allay anxieties, promote optimism and hope, contribute toward realistic planning, and offer psychological support and practical guidance to parents of the children involved.

A questionnaire was administered at mid-year (July, 1973) to which parents were asked to respond anonymously to a series of questions, many of which were open-ended. In December, as the first program year was drawing to a close, the same questionnaire was again administered. Since the anonymity of respondents was assured and maintained, it was not possible to distinguish between the observations of those new to the program and those who had been involved from the inception of Project HEED.

A total of fourteen parents (usually the mother, occasionally the father, grandmother, or other principal caregiver) responded. These were the parents who were in the program at the time the final assessment was made. The first set of questions elicited their general reactions to various aspects of the program and their participation in it. Their responses are summarized in Table V.

Parents of three children who participated during its first year dropped from the program for various reasons. In one instance a father who had been bringing his child opted to complete his own high school education, making it impossible for him to continue in HEED. A mother of another child resumed her teaching career and withdrew her son, while another dropped out suddenly, apparently in a panic concerning an impending hospitalization. The remaining nineteen continued to participate in HEED as long as the staff felt that this program was appropriate for them.

As Table V suggests, the parents expressed a sense of satisfaction with the general design of the project in terms of those components noted (i.e. parent participation in and observation of the classroom, parent meetings and contact with HEED staff). All felt their child had made *much* or *very much* progress, with approximately two thirds of those responding indicating that "very much" progress had been made. All but one indicated that their efforts at home in helping their child had been aided by participation in HEED.

Three parents revealed that they did not find being in the classroom setting with their own child and other children helpful, although two of these enjoyed the experience. Since such participation was considered an important aspect of the project, further discussion would seem indicated relative to the usefulness and helpfulness of a parent assuming a teacher role, why it might not be working out as anticipated, and under what circumstances this intent should be modified.

Although all said they enjoyed both parent meetings and classroom observation, one did not find the meetings and another the observation particularly helpful. The remainder were nearly equally divided for both activities in terms of whether it was "very helpful" or merely "helpful."

The remainder of the questionnaire was intended to encour-

TABLE V
Parent Questionnaire Responses
(December, 1973)

1. Understood purpose of HEED	Well 12	Somewhat 2		Not at All	0
2. Believed child has progressed	Very Much 9	Much 5	Some 0	Not at All	0
3. Believe (parent's) being in classroom was	Very Helpful	7	Enjoyable, but not Helpful		2
	Helpful	4	Neither enjoyable nor helpful		1
4. Believe (parent's) observing classroom was	Very Helpful	6	Enjoyable, but not Helpful		1
	Helpful	7	Neither enjoyable nor helpful		0
5. Believe parent meetings were	Very Helpful	5	Enjoyable, but not Helpful		1
	Helpful	8	Neither enjoyable nor helpful		0
6. Believe HEED was helpful aiding (parent's) work with child at home	Much	11	Little		1
	Some	2	No		0
7. (Parent) learned from	HEED staff	13	Observing		8
	Other parents	9			

age parents to elaborate on their evaluative judgments, to raise specific questions or criticism, and to offer suggestions. Their responses reflected, in general, great satisfaction with HEED. If any particular area could be specifically singled out as most appreciated by parents, it would appear to be the opportunity to converse and interact with, and to learn from, the HEED staff. Observations relating to this theme ranged from appreciation of the staff's desire to communicate insights and techniques to parents in individual informal discussions to more structured presentations by staff at parent meetings. Observations also included references to the learning gained through observing staff at work with their children, and several individuals noted the apparent conscientiousness and, even more, sincere interest in the children manifest in the way these professionals worked with their children.

A few specific criticisms and suggestions were offered, including the need for more than two sessions each week. These also included suggestions that more time with the professional staff would be helpful. Many parents noted areas of growth in their child or in themselves which they attributed to HEED. The former observations included the child's ability to separate and to interact with peers, as well as growth in specific areas such as language acquisition, ambulation, and greater independence. Areas of self-growth specifically noted included gains in their own ability to cope with the problems of caring for a handicapped child and in understanding the growth needs and patterns of young children.

As observers of the HEED classroom, nearly all parents appear to have liked what they saw: a varied program of appropriately selected activity directed toward the individual needs and developmental readiness of each child, carried out by competent yet relaxed, warm, and caring professionals.

CONCLUSIONS RELATED TO HEED OBJECTIVES

When Project HEED was conceived, several general objectives thought to be applicable for most children and parents who would participate were formulated and their rationale presented. These were subsequently stated in somewhat more precise terms and the means to be used to determine program effectiveness in attaining each was described. As has been noted, however, these objectives became meaningful only when translated into much more specific, behavioral, and operational terms for each individual child and parent.

In this section, the major objectives are reviewed and a statement made which is intended to summarize some conclusions and inferences drawn from the data presented in preceding sections. A set of recommendations for program modifications is then offered, some of which have already been instituted, and for continuation of the program, assuming that financial support for its continuance will be available.

The first set of objectives pertained to the children. Each begins with the stem: *The child will....*, indicating that the objectives relate to child accomplishments enabled by staff rather than to staff activities alone. For example, to state that an adult will teach a child color discrimination does not necessarily ensure that the child will be able to discriminate colors. These objectives, then, rest on assessments of children's behavior change previously documented.

Objectives (Children)

1. *Accomplish age-appropriate developmental tasks; body mastery; sense of competence; exploration of environment; independence (individuation and autonomy)*

That mother-child separation was accomplished with relative ease by nearly all children (and their mothers) indicates in itself a progression toward autonomy and individuation. Marked gains which were nearly universal were indicated in the four dimensions of the Teacher's Periodic Checklist, especially for those children whose overall intellectual functioning was at a two to three-year-old level, the period during which strivings for autonomy are anticipated. Considerably less progress was made by those children functioning at a substantially younger level.

In both the physical therapy assessment (functional age) and the self-awareness and body mastery dimension of the Teacher's Periodic Checklist, greater functional control over body movements and awareness of body-image and self were reflected. Increases in these two areas were more striking than any other. The relatively slower progress in the Activities of Daily Living dimension of the occupational therapy assessment, however, suggests that much growth is yet needed in terms of mastery of body functions and that perhaps this aspect should receive greater emphasis.

2. *Achieve self-awareness and positive self-evaluation.*

The teacher's observations, both reflected in her ratings for self-awareness and body mastery on the TPC and through the team's observations recorded in the Daily Record, suggested that staff generally perceived most HEED children to have progressed in this respect. Primarily impressionistic and parent-report data must suffice to permit the conclusion that positive self-feelings and a greater sense of competence and worth were associated with HEED participation.

3. *Achieve readiness for nursery school and therapy program of agency.*

HEED was not conceived primarily to be a readiness program for nursery school although, as of January, 1974, ten HEED "graduates" had moved into the regular nursery school program. As was suggested in earlier discussion, greater provision for one-to-one assistance and greater parent participation in the nursery school might serve to make this transition more natural and accomplished more optimally. For some children, too, continued participation in a HEED-type program would be a more viable alternative in view of severely limited functioning.

4. *Attain security regarding separation.*

The matter of separation was notably successfully handled through the HEED program, as was observed with reference to Objective 1. That parents could continue to be accessible, either in the classroom or the observation room where they were visible to children, facilitated this process.

5. *Gain experience in a peer setting.*

For many children HEED represented their first peer interactive experience and was an important prelude to entrance into nursery school and, eventually, into regular or special education programs. Informal observations and impressions and parent reports tended to substantiate the TPC ratings of important gains in social adaptation.

6. *Gain experience with adults in a teaching role.*

Again, as with peer interaction, these experiences did in fact take place. It was evident that, with exceptions in Group III described in Chapter 14, children in HEED did establish meaningful relationships with the teacher, physical therapist, and teaching assistant, with whom they regularly interacted. The ability of most HEED children to respond to group instruction and therapeutic sessions administered by the speech pathologist on a staggered schedule basis was also observed.

   7. *Attain cognitive and linguistic learning: symbolic play; receptive and expressive language functions; imitation; object permanence; causality; object schemas; basic form; size, color, and relational concepts.*

Language age gain scores which, as was indicated previously, were statistically significant for the group as a whole and even more pronounced for particular subgroups, revealed important development in abilities to take in messages and to use speech communicatively and language in the service of thought. The case studies presented in Chapter 13 illustrate instances in which major gains were made in this respect. That language progress occurred, in most instances, is unquestionable. However, to what extent specific components of the HEED program brought about particular gains on the part of individual children must rely on analysis of individual records as they were developed formatively.

In terms of cognitive attainments, the program focus was dual: (1) to provide the "building blocks for learning" of the sensorimotor period, which might have been imperfectly acquired due to the physical limitations on motor function, and (2) to move from these key areas of imitation, object permanence, and physical causality into true representational thought, as reflected in deferred imitation, imaginative play, concepts of time and space, and related learning. Both impressionistic observation and TPC ratings increases suggest a degree of success in such areas as these, again noting the serious limitations of attainment possible among children in Group III.

The second set of general objectives pertained to the parents. Program impact on parents can be inferred not only on the basis of rating scale data reported earlier but also from the consistency of participation revealed in the attendance data. Again parent objectives began with the stem: *To enable the parent to. . . .*

Objectives (Parents)

1. *View their children as learners and themselves as teachers, as well as mothers.*

Several items from both the caseworker's evaluation and the Parent Checklist were directed toward this concept, that one important facet of the parent-child bond, and in particular the mother-child bond, is a dyadic teaching and learning relationship. The caseworker's ratings and questionnaire responses both suggested that a greater awareness of the learning capabilities and accomplishments of their child was achieved by many parents and that they were able to see the possibilities for their own greater success in facilitating development. The parents tended to attribute this to the program, especially their contacts with the program staff from whom they felt much had been learned. Although it is difficult to objectively assess, it is certain that the facilitating role of the caseworker herself is promoting both a degree of realistic hope and positive action on the part of HEED parents was of paramount importance.

2. *Imitate and learn from role models provided by teachers and therapists ways of interacting with their children which may enhance development.*

This objective relates to the first in a reciprocal fashion. The opportunity for modeling and learning through other means is a necessary but not sufficient condition for parents to extend the HEED impact into the home setting. A degree of self-confidence, as well as awareness of the possibilities which may be employed, is necessary. Nearly all parents did indicate that they had learned substantially from HEED staff and had profited from their opportunities to work with the staff in directly assisting their children.

The very few exceptions, however, suggest the need to continue to give special attention to this aspect of the program and to the differential needs and readiness levels among parents for such approaches as observation, practicing behaviors demonstrated by staff models, didactic learning, direct vs. indirect guidance, and group discussion.

3. *Express and share their feelings as parents of handicapped children, thus gaining a sense of solidarity.*

The HEED parents conveyed through the Parent Questionnaire a sense of appreciation for the mutual associations with other parents gained through the program. Both casual observation of the many informal dialogues held spontaneously by parents and more conscious appraisal of their mutual interaction in the context of parent group meetings suggested that, for most participating parents, this objective had been successfully achieved.

4. *Gain a greater sense of their ability to foster their children's learning and development in spite of handicaps.*

The HEED program offered a balance of educative and supportive assistance to which nearly all parents appear to have responded, albeit in varying ways and to varying degrees. Many parents expressed great concerns about such everyday crises as those often involved in mealtimes. Through mutual sharing of experiences and ideas, as well as guidance from HEED staff, most parents appear to have gained reinforcement and confidence concerning their own ability to help their child at home. Many parents seemed to be impressed with the busy, yet very warm and happy atmosphere of learning created in the HEED classroom and gained enjoyment and satisfaction from their own participation in it.

RECOMMENDATIONS

The basic philosophy of HEED appears to have been demonstrated viable, on the basis of substantial gains made by children, parent expressions of satisfaction and generally positive feedback, and the experience of HEED staff in functioning as an interdisciplinary integrated team. The HEED model would appear to be appropriate not only for handicapped children in the eighteen through thirty-six month age range, but also possibly for older handicapped children and for young children with developmental problems other than a physical disability (mental retardation, emotional disturbance). For staff the HEED experience provided a source of ideas for alternative programming for these groups, both within the Agency's regular program and in the community.

For children such as those who participated in HEED during its first year, 1973, there must be alternative programming strategies available. For those children with severe general retardation and/or sensory impairment and neurological dysfunction, the program must be quite different from that for the handicapped child of normal or near normal intellectual ability or without pronounced sensory deficits.

As HEED evolved, its participants seemed to fall into one of these two general categories, despite the wide range of individual differences within each, and two discrete programs were developed. The sensory group alternates basic sensory stimulation with relaxation and emphasizes critical basic areas such as feeding. For this group, a one-to-one adult-child ration is essential for most components of such a program, and staffing and parent participation variations have been experimented with in order to permit this. The goals, activities, assessment procedures, and the physical surroundings themselves must be radically different from those used successfully with the more able and less seriously impaired youngsters, regardless of chronological age differences.

It was still hoped that fathers could become more closely involved in the project, although one or two fathers were principal participants, rather than their wives. Possibly the addition of a male caseworker to the staff might encourage some fathers to take more active part.

Greater explicit emphasis may need to be placed on Activities of Daily Living, i.e. consciously teaching the children aspects of self-care important both to their general competence and growth and to their sense of autonomy and self-worth.

It was also concluded that every effort must continue to be made to maximize the meaningful participation of parents in various aspects of the program including guided observation, participation in the classroom, and participation in group meetings. It would be desirable to extend the guidance and follow-up emphasis into the home itself in order to ensure maximum carry-over.

The long range effects of early intervention through such programs as this, obviously, cannot be ascertained for years to come. Whether Project HEED has, in fact, made a difference in terms of the physical, intellectual, emotional, and social development of the children it has served will not be immediately known. Their progress must be followed over time.

Preliminary findings, however, offer strong support for the position that very young children with physical handicaps do manifest pronounced needs in the psychosocial and cognitive spheres, to which comprehensive and integrated intervention may successfully be addressed. Possibly, programs similar to HEED might be undertaken with even younger children.

Project HEED has served a truly generative function. It is hoped that this is primarily true of the direct service provided those children and families who were its participants during its first year of operation. Hopefully, their experiences in the program have been a source of new hope, courage, knowledge, and skills, and the impact of HEED on the lives of these children will have far-reaching consequences.

The program has been generative, too, in the sense of the vast learning opportunity it provided for HEED staff. The skills of each staff member, both in providing direct service to clients and in maximizing the benefits of that service through an integrated team approach, were immeasurably enhanced. Each aspect of the program, including its emphasis on the parent-child relationship, integration of special therapies within a nursery classroom, communications among an interdisciplinary team, and all others, was a source of continuing challenge and constantly fresh insight.

It is hoped that the impact of Project HEED will extend beyond the limitations of the small number of children and families such programs are able to serve directly. In addition to the need for continued progress in the field of medicine which will hopefully lead to many additional significant breakthroughs in the search for ameliorative, curative, and preventive means, there is a great need for imaginative, skillful, and sensitive facilitators of development for young children who are born with or incur early in life a physically handicapping condition. If through Project HEED new ideas and viable techniques are demonstrated and shared with others in the helping professions and the community at large, it will have made a significant contribution.

BIBLIOGRAPHY

Ainsworth, Mary D.: Patterns of attachment behavior shown by the infant in interaction with his mother. *Merrill-Palmer Quarterly, 10*:51, 1964.

Anderson, Ruth, Miles, Madeline, and Matheny, Patricia: *Communicative Evaluation Chart from Infancy to Five Years*. Cambridge, Educators' Publishing Service, 1963.

Apgar, Virginia, and Beck, Joan: *Is My Baby All Right? A Guide to Birth Defects*. New York, Trident, 1972.

Ayres, Jean: *Sensory Integration and Learning Disorders*. Los Angeles, Western Psychological Services, 1972.

Barker, Roger: *Adjustment to Physical Handicap and Illness: A Survey of The Social Psychology of Physique and Disability*. New York, Social Science Research Council, 1953.

Bettelheim, Bruno: *The Empty Fortress*. New York, Macmillan-Free Press, 1967.

Bloom, Benjamin S.: *Stability and Change in Human Characteristics*. New York, Wiley, 1964.

Bower, Eli M.: Three rivers of significance to education. In Bower, Eli M., and Hollister, William G. (Eds.): *Behavioral Science Frontiers in Education*. New York, Wiley, 1967.

Bowlby, John: *Maternal Care and Mental Health*. New York, Shocken, 1966.

Bruner, Jerome S.: *Toward a Theory of Instruction*. New York, Norton, 1966.

Buhler, Charlotte: *The First Year of Life*. New York, John Day, 1930.

Bzoch, Kenneth R., and League, Richard: *The Bzoch-League Receptive-Expressive Emergent Language Scale for the Measurement of Language Skills in Infancy*. Gainesville, Language Education Division, Computer Management Corporation, 1970.

Caplan, Gerald (Ed.): *Prevention of Mental Disorders in Children*. New York, Basic Books, 1961.

Casler, Lawrence: The effects of extra tactile stimulation on a group of institutionalized infants. *Genet Psychol Monogr, 71*:137, 1965.

Cattell, Psyche: *The Measurement of Intelligence of Infants and Young Children*. New York, Psychological Corporation, 1947.

Crabtree, Margaret: *The Houston Test for Language Development*. Houston, Houston Test Company, 1958.

Cruickshank, William M., and Johnson, Orville: *Education of Exceptional Children and Youth*. Englewood Cliffs, Prentice-Hall, 1967.

Dennis, Wayne, and Najarian, P.: Infant development under environmental handicap. *Psychol Monogr, 71*:436, 1957.

Deno, Evelyn: *Instructional Alternatives for Exceptional Children*. Arlington, The Council for Exceptional Children, 1973.

289

DiLeo, Joseph H.: *Young Children and Their Drawings*. New York, Brunner and Mazel, 1970.

Doll, Edgar A.: *Measurement of Social Competence*. Minneapolis, American Guidance Service, 1953.

Doll, Edgar A.: *Preschool Attainment Record: A Preschool Scale of Development*. Minneapolis, American Guidance Service, 1966.

Dolphin, James E., and Cruickshank, William M.: The figure-background relationship in children with cerebral palsy. *J Clin Psychol,* 7:228, 1951.

Elkind, David: *Children and Adolescents: Interpretive Essays on Jean Piaget*. London, Oxford, 1970.

Erikson, Erik H.: *Childhood and Society*. New York, Norton, 1950.

Fantz, Robert L., and Nevis, Sonia: Pattern preferences and perceptual-cognitive development in early infancy. *Merrill-Palmer Quarterly, 13*:77, 1967.

Finnie, Nancie: *Handling the Young Cerebral Palsied Child at Home*. New York, Dutton, 1970.

Fiorentino, Mary R.: *Reflex Testing Methods for Evaluating C.N.S. Development*. Springfield, Thomas, 1973.

Flavell, John: *The Developmental Psychology of Jean Piaget*. Princeton, Van Nostrand, 1963.

Fraiberg, Selma: *The Magic Years*. New York, Scribner, 1959.

Fraiberg, Selma, Siegel, B. L., and Gibson, R.: The role of sound in the searching behavior of a blind infant. *Psychoanal Study Child, 21*:327, 1966.

Freedheim, Donald K.: Individuality of intellectual development. *Journal of the American Physical Therapy Association, 46*:149, 1966.

Furth, Hans G.: Research with the deaf: Implications for language and cognition. *Psychol Bull, 61*:145, 1964.

Gesell, Arnold L., and Amatruda, C. S.: *Developmental Diagnosis*. New York, Hoeber, 1941.

Gillette, Harriet E.: *Systems of Therapy in Cerebral Palsy*. Springfield, Thomas, 1969.

Ginsburg, Herbert, and Opper, Sylvia: *Piaget's Theory of Intellectual Development: An Introduction*. Englewood Cliffs, Prentice-Hall, 1969.

Hebb, Donald O.: *The Organization of Behavior*. New York, Wiley, 1949.

Hunt, Joseph McVicker: *Intelligence and Experience*. New York, Ronald, 1961.

Inhelder, Barbel, and Piaget, Jean: *The Child's Concept of Space*. New York, Norton, 1967.

Inhelder, Barbel, and Piaget, Jean: *The Early Growth of Logic in The Child*. New York, Norton, 1964.

Inhelder, Barbel, and Piaget, Jean: *The Psychology of The Child*. New York, Basic Books, 1969.

Isaacs, Susan: *Intellectual Growth in Young Children*. New York, Shocken, 1971.

Kamii, Constance: An application of Piaget's theory to the conceptualization of a preschool curriculum. In Parker, Ronald W. (Ed.): *The Preschool in Action*. Boston, Allyn and Bacon, 1973.

Keats, Sidney: *Cerebral Palsy*. Springfield, Thomas, 1973.

Kellog, Rhoda: *The Psychology of Children's Art*. New York, Random House, 1967.

Kessen, William: Sucking and looking: two organized congenital patterns of behavior in the human newborn. In Stevenson, Harold W., Hess, Edward H., and Rheingold, Harriet L. (Eds.): *Early Behavior: Comparative and Developmental Approaches*. New York, Wiley, 1967.

Kessler, Jane W.: *Psychopathology of Childhood*. Englewood Cliffs, Prentice-Hall, 1966.

Knoblock, Hilda, Pasamanick, Benjamin, and Sherard, Earl: *A Developmental Screening Inventory*. Columbus, 1954.

Knott, Margaret, and Voss, Dorothy E.: *Proprioceptive Neuromuscular Facilitation*. New York, Harper and Row, 1968.

Lowenfeld, Victor, and Brittain, W. L.: *Creative and Mental Growth*, 4th ed. New York, Macmillan, 1964.

Mahler, Margaret S.: On early infantile psychoses: The symbiotic and autistic syndromes. *Journal of Academic Child Psychiatry, 4*:554, 1965.

Mahler, Margaret S.: Thoughts about development and individuation. *Psychoanal Study Child, 18*:307, 1962.

McGraw, Myrtle B.: *The Neuromuscular Maturation of The Human Infant*. New York and London, Hafner, 1963.

Nelson, Waldo E., Vaughan, Victor C., III, and McKay, R. James: *Textbook of Pediatrics*. Philadelphia, Saunders, 1969.

Ojemann, Ralph: Investigation of the effects of teaching understanding and appreciation of behavior dynamics. In Caplan, Gerald (Ed.): *Prevention of Mental Disorders in Children*. New York, Basic Books, 1961.

Page, Dorothy: Neuromuscular reflex therapy as an approach to patient care. *Am J Phys Med, 46*:816, 1967.

Phelps, William M.: Recent significant trends in the case of cerebral palsy. *South Med J, 38*:132, 1946.

Piaget, Jean: *The Origins of Intelligence in Children*. New York, Norton, 1952.

Piaget, Jean: *Play, Dreams and Imitation in Childhood*. New York, Norton, 1962.

Piaget, Jean: *Six Psychological Studies*. New York, Random House, 1967.

Pines, Maya: *Revolution in Learning*. New York, Harper and Row, 1966.

Pinneau, Samuel R.: A critique on the articles by Margaret Ribble. *Child Dev, 21*:203, 1950.

Plank, Emma: Preparing children for surgery. *Ohio State Med J, 59*:809, 1963.

Plank, Emma: *Working with Children in Hospitals*. Cleveland, Western Reserve University Press, 1962.

Powledge, Fred: *To Change A Child: A Report on The Institute for Developmental Studies*. Chicago, Qudrangle, 1967.

Rogers, Carl R.: A theory of therapy, personality, and interpersonal relationships, as developed in the client-centered framework. In Koch, Sigmund (Ed.): *Psychology: A Study of A Science*. New York, Wiley, vol. III, pp. 184-256.

Rohwer, William C., Jr.: Cognitive and perceptual development in children. Paper presented at the Conference on Manpower Preparation for Handicapped Young Children, Washington, D.C., December 9 and 10, 1971.

Sattler, Jerome M. and Anderson, N. E.: Peabody Picture Vocabulary Test, Stanford-Binet, and modified Stanford-Binet with normal and cerebral palsied preschool children. *Journal of Special Education*, 7:119, 1973.

Semans, Sarah: The Bobath concept in treatment of neurological disorders. *Am J Phys Med*, 46:732, 1967.

Sigel, Irving E.: The attainment of concepts. In Hoffman, Martin H. and Hoffman, Lois W. (Eds.): *Review of Child Development Research*. New York, Russell Sage, vol. I, pp. 209-248.

Silberman, Charles E.: *Crisis in The Classroom: The Remaking of American Education*. New York, Random House, 1970.

Small, Gloria: *Environment and Early Education: An Experimental Course*. Cleveland, Case Western Reserve University Press, 1973.

Smilansky, Sara: *The Effects of Sociodramatic Play on Disadvantaged Preschool Children*. New York, Wiley, 1968.

Spitz, Rene A.: Hospitalism: an inquiry into the genesis of psychiatric conditions in early childhood. *Psychoanal Study Child*, 1:53, 1945.

Spock, Benjamin, and Lerrigo, Marion O.: *Caring for Your Disabled Child*. New York, Macmillan, 1965.

Stockmeyer, Shirley A.: An interpretation of the approach of Rood to the treatment of neuromuscular dysfunction. *Am J Phys Med*, 46:900, 1967.

Strauss, Alfred A., and Lehtinen, Laura E.: *Psychopathology and Education of The Brain-injured Child*. New York, Grune and Stratton, 1947.

Sullivan, Harry S.: *The Interpersonal Theory of Psychiatry*. New York, Norton, 1953.

Telford, Charles W. and Sawrey, James M.: *The Exceptional Individual: Psychological and Educational Aspects*. Englewood Cliffs, Prentice-Hall, 1967.

Tyler, Nancy S.: A steriognosis test for screening tactile sensation. *Am J Occup ther*, 26:256, 1972.

Uzgiris, Ina C., and Hunt, Joseph, McV.: *A Scale of Infant Psychological Development*. (Mimeographed). Urbana, University of Illinois, 1964.

Weikart, David, Deloria, D., Lawser, Sara, and Weigerink, Ronald: *Longitudinal Results of The Ypsilanti Perry Preschool Project*. Washington, U. S. Department of Health, Education and Welfare, Office of Education, Bureau of Research, 1970.

Wenar, Charles: The effects of a motor handicap on personality, II: The effects on integrative ability. *Child Dev*, 25:287, 1954.

White, Robert W.: Motivation reconsidered: The concept of competence. *Psychol rev*, 66:297, 1959.

Wohlwill, Joachim: From perception to inference. In Kessen, William, and Kuhlman, Clementina (Eds.): *Thought in The Young Child*. Monographs of the Society for Research in Child Development, 1962, Whole No. 83.

Wolff, Peter H.: The causes, controls, and organization of behavior in the neonate. *Psychol Issues*, 5:7, 1966.

APPENDIX A
GOALS AND PROGRESS RECORD FORM

PROJECT HEED

DATE _____

NAME _____

	LONG-RANGE GOALS	IMMEDIATE GOALS	ACTIVITIES	PROGRESS
P.T.				
ED.				
SPEECH				
O.T.				
S.W.				

APPENDIX B
EDUCATION ASSESSMENT INSTRUMENTS

TEACHER'S DAILY REPORT

CHILD _____
DATE _____
TEACHER _____

1. Separation _____
2. Peer Interaction _____
   _____
   _____

3. Teacher Interaction _____
   _____

4. Motor Activity Initiated _____
   _____

5. Imitative Behavior _____
   _____

6. General Affect _____
7. Mother-Child Interaction _____
   _____

8. Other Comments

Problem Solving Behavior

Activity	New or Familiar	Affect	P.S. Strategy	Verbalization

TEACHER'S CHECKLIST

O-Never
1-Rarely
2-Often
3-Consistently

I. Self-Awareness and Body Mastery
  A. Self-Awareness
    1. Recognizes own name   _____
    2. Vocally identifies self   _____
    3. Recognizes full-view mirror reflection of self   _____

4. Recognizes own photograph when it is presented together with photograph of another child
5. Recognizes own photograph when it is presented together with several photographs of other children _____
6. Asserts ownership of toys or other items _____
7. Can correctly express whether he is a boy or girl _____

B. Recognition of Body Parts
  1. Can point to or identify head _____
  2. Can point to or identify eyes _____
  3. Can point to or identify nose _____
  4. Can point to or identify mouth _____
  5. Can point to or identify ears _____
  6. Can point to or identify hands _____
  7. Can point to or identify arms _____
  8. Can point to or identify legs _____
  9. Can point to or identify feet _____
 10. Can point to or identify hair _____
 11. Can point to or identify teeth _____
 12. Can point to or identify finger-nails _____
 13. Can point to or identify tummy _____
 14. Can point to or identify shoulders _____

C. Body Mastery
  1. Communicates need to toilet _____
  2. Can feed self a cookie _____
  3. Can drink milk from a cup _____
  4. Can use tissue, handkerchief, napkin _____
  5. Initiates gross motor activity in play _____
  6. Initiates fine motor activity in play _____
  7. Participates or assists in removing outer clothes _____
  8. Participates or assists in donning outer clothing _____

II. Exploration of Environment
  1. Will seek desired object temporarily hidden from view. _____
  2. Will solicit adult assistance. _____
  3. Enjoys manipulating play materials. _____
  4. Becomes absorbed in play. _____
  5. Plays with many diverse toys and materials. _____
  6. Uses familiar objects for new purposes. _____
  7. Within limits imposed by handicap, moves about in physical space. _____
  8. Play behavior with, for example, blocks is purposive. _____
  9. Uses objects as tools in achieving own purposes (e.g., a stick as extension of arm; a chair to stand on.) _____
 10. Enjoys new experiences. _____
 11. Enjoys investigating a new toy. _____
 12. Will persevere in problem-solving with toys, puzzles, etc. _____
 13. Reflects pattern in block building. _____

III. Social Adaptation
  1. Separates readily from mother. _____
  2. Appears happy and content. _____

    3. Shows awareness of peers as individuals.   ———

    4. Engages in parallel play.   ———

    5. Can recognize the name of and correctly identify at least one peer.   ———

    6. Initiates interaction with peers.   ———

    7. Initiates interaction with adult other then parent.   ———

    8. Vocally refers to one or more peers as individuals.   ———

    9. Will follow a simple verbal instruction.

    10. Joins in group activities such as singing, finger plays, rhythmics.   ———

IV. Cognitive Skills

    1. Engages in symbolic (representational) play.   ———

    2. Vocally narrates own play.   ———

    3. Will imitate an adult behavior when directed.   ———

    4. Will imitate an adult behavior spontaneously.   ———

    5. Will imitate a peer behavior when asked by adult.   ———

    6. Will imitate a peer behavior spontaneously.   ———

    7. When presented two objects differing in size, can select the *big* object.   ———

    8. When presented two objects differing in size, can select the *little* object.   ———

    9. Will pursue a desired object when it is hidden from his view (placed behind screen by adult).   ———

    10. Will pursue a desired object when it is successively moved behind first one screen, then other.   ———

    11. Makes reference to or shows recognition of named objects not present or in view.   ———

    12. Builds blocks vertically.   ———

    13. Correctly discrimates squares, circular and triangular forms in using a form toy.   ———

    14. Can complete 1-piece formboard puzzle using trial-and-error manipulations.   ———

    15. When presented with three rubber balls (large) and three other items of similar size, can place balls in a container.   ———

    16. Can complete ball task when balls are of very different size.   ———

    17. Can identify a desired object.   ———

    18. Will intentionally repeat a play sequence several times.   ———

    19. Recalls location of specific toys and other items.   ———

    20. Can match color.   ———

    21. Spatial Relationships: Can distinguish

        a. up   ———

        b. down   ———

        c. in   ———

        d. out   ———

        e. over   ———

        f. under   ———

        g. through   ———

        h. around   ———

APPENDIX C
PHYSICAL THERAPY ASSESSMENT INSTRU-MENTS

MOTOR DEVELOPMENT TEST*

NAME _____

DIAGNOSIS_____

Scoring:

   A = Beginning activity, but unable to complete.

   B = Accomplishes activity with some assistance.

   C = Accomplishes activity, but in more than average time, or in an awkward manner.

   D = Accomplishes activity within normal limits and within average time.

   M = Patient has reached maximum due to disability.

TEST RESULTS

							TEST DATES
Basal Age							
Equivalent level of normal accomplishment (Composite score of D)							
Functional level of accomplishment (Composite score of C&D							
Level of highest accomplishment							

*Adapted from the C.P. Dept., West Haverstraw, N.Y. State Rehab. Hosp. and Fernald State School, Waltham, Mass.

Age Level	Items	Date			
3 Months					
Prone	1. Head compensates when held in ventral suspension				
	2. Lifts head when resting on forearms				
	3. On verge of rolling to supine.				
	4. Head rotates and extends				
Supine	5. Symmetrical hand and arm posture.				
	6. Rolls part way to side				
Supported	7. Slight head lag when pulled to sitting				
Sitting	8. Head steady, lumbar curve				
Supported Standing	9. Bears small fraction of weight on legs briefly				
6 Months					
Prone	10. Lifts arm with stimulation				
	11. Rolls to supine				
	12. Legs and arms extended, weight on hands				
	13. Circular pivoting				
Supine	14. Lifts head				
	15. Rolls to prone				
Sitting	16. Lifts head and assists in pull to sitting				
	17. Sits momentarily, leaning on hands				
	18. Active in supported sitting				
9 Months					
Prone	19. Assumes hand-knee crawling position				
	20. Pulls self along floor on stomach or creeps				
Sitting	21. Sits indefinitely				
	22. Prone to sitting, sitting to prone				
Standing	23. Pulls to standing at furniture				
	24. Lowers to floor with support				
1 Year					
Posture and	25. Assumes and maintains kneeling balance				
Locomotion	26. Knee walks				
	27. Pivots in sitting				
	28. Cruises				
	29. Climbs on furniture				
	30. Walks with one hand held				

Age Level	Items	Date			
15 Months					
Posture	31. Walks alone, seldom falls				
and	32. Walks alone a few steps				
Locomotion	33. Crawls or hitches upstairs				
18 Months					
Posture	34. Walks alone, seldom falls				
and	35. Upstairs with one hand held				
Locomotion	36. Seats self in small chair				
21 Months					
Locomotion	37. Upstairs holding one rail				
	38. Downstairs, with one hand held				
	39. Squates in play				
2 Years					
Locomotion	40. Runs fairly well				
	41. Up and down stairs alone, one step at a time				
	42. Kicks in standing				
3 Years					
	43. Walks on tip toes				
	44. Runs on toes				
	45. Rides tricycle				
	46. Jumps on both feet				
	47. Upstairs, alternating feet				
	48. Momentary one foot standing				
4 Years					
	49. Downstairs, alternating feet				
	50. One foot standing balance 4-8 sec.				
	51. Skips on one foot				

REFLEX RESPONSES

NAME: _____

B.D. _____

THERAPIST _____

DATE: _____

REFLEX LEVEL	REFLEX	+ or −	POSITIVE REFLEX REACTION	COMMENT
I. Spinal Normal: Birth—	1. Flexor Withdrawal Supine—stimulate sole		Uncontrolled flex. stimulated leg	
2 mos	2. Extensor Thrust Supine-one leg ext. one flexed—stimulate flexed leg's sole		Uncontrolled extension stimulated leg	
	3. Crossed Extension Supine—one leg flex—one leg ext. Flex extended leg		Opposite leg will extend	
II. Brain Stem Normal up to	4. Asymmetrical Tonic Neck		Ext. face side, flexion opposite side	
4 to 6 months	5. Symmetrical Tonic Neck Prone over knee		Ventro-flex—Uppers flex, lowers ext. Dorsiflex-Uppers ext., lowers flex	
	6. Tonic Labyrinthine Prone		Increase in flexor tone	

Age	Item	Response
	7. Tonic Labyrinthine Supine	Increase in extensor tone
	8. Associated Reactions Squeeze object	Mirroring of opposite limb +/ or in tone in other parts of body
	9. Positive Supporting Reaction—Bounce several times on soles	Increase in extensor tone
	10. Negative Supporting Reaction—Bounce on soles then hold in space	Increase in flexor tone
III. MIDBRAIN Birth—6 mos	11. Neck Righting Supine rotate head to one side	Body rotates as a whole
6 mos—life	12. Body righting acting on body—Supine—rotate head to one side	Segmental rotation
6 mos—8 mos life	13. LABYRINTHINE RIGHTING Blindfolded in space	Head rights to normal position
6 mos—8 mos life	14. OPTICAL RIGHTING Hold in space	Head rights to normal position
6 mos—life	15. AMPHIBIAN REACTION Prone—lift pelvis one side	Flexion arm, hip, knee, same side

REFLEX RESPONSES (Continued)

REFLEX LEVEL	REFLEX	+ or –	POSITIVE REFLEX REACTION	COMMENT
IV. AUTOMATIC MOVEMENT Birth—4 to 6 mos	16. MORO		Abd.-ext. reaction	
6 mos to 2½ yrs.	17. LANDAU Prone in space—raise head		Spine and legs extend	
6 mos—life	18. PROTECTIVE EXT. THRUST Suspend-move suddenly towards floor		Immediate ext. of arms with abd. and ext. of fingers	
V. CORTICAL Equilibrium Reactions 6 mos 8 mos 10—12 mos 10 mos	19. Prone-supine 20. Four foot kneeling 21. Sitting 22. Kneel standing } Tilt to one side		Righting of head and thorax, abd—ext. of arm and leg on raised side, protective re-action on lowered side.	
15—18 mos thru life	23. Hopping Standing—move to side, front, back		Righting of head and thorax, hopping steps to maintain equilibrium	

APPENDIX E
CASEWORK ASSESSMENT INSTRUMENT

CASEWORK'S ASSESSMENT

DEGREE OF PROBLEM

FUNCTION
- Major Problem
- Needs Improvement
- Adequate

FEELINGS RECOGNIZE EXPRESS
- Not at All
- Some
- Well

ACCEPT OR DENY
- Not At All
- Some
- Adequate

MOVEMENT
- Considerable Progress
- Some Progress
- Fluctuations
- Unknown
- Not Relevant

ACCEPTANCE DENIAL CONTINUUM

1. Expresses recognition of child's handicap.
2. Labels child handicap.
3. Expresses recognition of child's current limits and capabilities.
4. Discusses experiences in handling strangers' looks or comments about handicapped child.
5. Responds to such looks or comments appropriately.
6. Able to interpret child's future as realistically as possible.
7. Able to interpret child's problem to family or friends.
8. Appropriateness of affect re child.
9. Discusses experience of first learning of child's problems.

307

CASEWORKER'S ASSESSMENT

DEGREE OF PROBLEM

FUNCTION	Major Problem
	Need Improvement
	Adequate
FEELINGS RECOGNIZE EXPRESS	Not at All
	Some
	Well
ACCEPT OR DENY	Not at All
	Some
	Adequate

MOVEMENT

- Considerable Progress
- Some Progress
- Fluctuation
- Regression or None
- Unknown
- Not Relevant

FEELINGS

10. Discusses own feelings of guilt about child's handicap.
11. Expresses anger about having a handicapped child.
12. Expresses feelings of anger and frustration at managing handicapped child.
13. Expresses feelings of anger and resentment at difficulty of parenting role in general.
14. Able to discuss specific problems of parenting.
15. Able to discuss with spouse feelings and concerns about child.
16. Able to discuss with spouse problems of family interaction.
17. Able to discuss experiences with hospitalization, surgery & bracing.
18. Recognizes and expresses depression/frustration—current.
19. Recognizes and expresses depression/frustration—past.
20. Appropriateness of affect (in general).

CASEWORKER'S ASSESSMENT

DEGREE OF PROBLEM / MOVEMENT			
FUNCTION	Major Problem		
	Needs Improvement		
	Adequate		
FEELINGS RECOGNIZE EXPRESS	Not at All		
	Some		
	Well		
ACCEPT OR DENY	Not At All		
	Some		
	Adequate		
MOVEMENT	Considerable Progress		
	Some Progress		
	Fluctuations		
	Unknown		
	Not Relevant		

FUNCTIONING WITH HANDICAPPED CHILD

21. Communication between parents about handling.
22. Able to provide home guidance based on medical and HEED advice.
23. Able to provide peer contact for child.
24. Able to provide for nutritional needs of child.
25. Able to provide for sleep needs of child.
26. Able to keep child clean.
27. Able to provide appropriate environmental stimulation for child.
28. Father interested and active as parent.
29. Able to provide child with opportunity for independent exploration.
30. Aware of child's likes and dislikes.
31. Handles child realistically in terms of his limits.
32. Able to see positive aspects of parental role.
33. Show ingenuity in providing care and/or equipment to meet special needs.
34. Usually shows acceptance rather than rejection in parenting role.
35. Able to separate from child.

CASEWORKER'S ASSESSMENT

	DEGREE OF PROBLEM																		
FUNCTION	Major Problem																		
	Needs Improvement																		
	Adequate																		
FEELINGS RECOGNIZE EXPRESS																			
	Not at All																		
	Some																		
	Well																		
ACCEPT OR DENY	Not At All																		
	Some																		
	Adequate																		
MOVEMENT	Considerable Progress																		
	Some Progress																		
	Fluctuations																		
	Unknown																		
	Not Relevant																		

FUNCTIONING IN REGARD TO PERSONAL RELATIONSHIPS

36. Constructive use of relationship with HEED personnel.
37. Constructive relationship with at least one other HEED parent.
38. Meaningful relationship with at least one member of a larger family.
39. Meaningful relationship with at least one friend.
40. Meaningful relationship with spouse.
41. Constructive use of HEED group meetings.
42. Constructive use of casework counseling.
43. Marital situation.
44. Functions generally free from debilitating depression.
45. Handling of other children.
46. Deals effectively with own needs in context of own individual situation.

HEED PARENT QUESTIONNAIRE

PARENT QUESTIONNAIRE

Instructions: Because HEED is a new program, it would be helpful to the HEED staff to have your ideas, comments and opinions about the HEED program. You *are not asked* to sign this questionnaire. Just put it in the plain envelope, which is attached, and place it in the box provided. It would be most helpful if you answer the questionnaire before discussing it with other parents. We appreciate your cooperation.

A. Circle the answer that best expresses your opinion:
  1. I understand the purposes of Project HEED:

   well   *somewhat*   *not at all*

  2. Since entering HEED my child has progressed:

   very little   *some*   *much*   *very much*

  3. Being in the classroom with my child and the other children has, for me, been:

   very helpful   *helpful*   *enjoyable but*   *neither enjoyable*
                                        not helpful   *not helpful*

  4. Observing the classroom has been:

   very helpful   *helpful*   *enjoyable but*   *neither enjoyable*
                                        not helpful   *nor helpful*

  5. I have found the parent meetings to be:

   very helpful   *helpful*   *enjoyable but*   *neither enjoyable*
                                        not helpful   *nor helpful*

  6. As far as helping me to help my child at home is concerned, HEED has been:

   not helpful   *of little help*   *of some help*   *of much help*

  7. I have learned from:

   HEED staff   *other parents* *observing the classroom*
   other (specify)

311

B. Please answer the following questions on the basis of your impressions of the HEED Project so far.

1. What do you think of your child's experience in HEED?

A. What has he especially benefited from?

B. What has he not benefited from?

2. What do you think is the most valuable part of your experience in HEED?

3. What don't you like about HEED?

4. How has the HEED staff been helpful? Could they be more helpful? How?

5. What kind of parent meetings do you like?

6. How could Project HEED be better?

7. What do other members of your family think about your child being in HEED?

C. Please list what you LIKE or DISLIKE of the following aspects of HEED

	LIKE	DISLIKE
1. Parents in the classroom		
2. HEED schedule		
3. Conferences with staff		
4. Children's activities		
5. Parent meetings		
6. Informal contacts with parents		
7. Observing the classroom		
8. Caseworker conferences		
9. Staff evaluations by teacher, psychologist, speech pathologist, physical therapist and occupational therapist		

D. Any other comments about HEED:
(use back of sheet)

APPENDIX G
PLAN VIEW OF HEED CLASSROOM

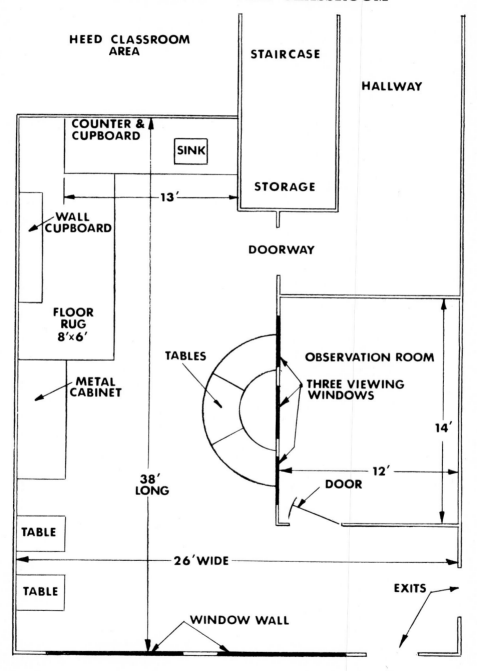

INDEX

A

Accident, as etiological agent, 15
Achondroplasia, 3, 4, 13
Activities of daily living, 153, 170-172
Ainsworth, Mary B., 81
Ames, Louise B., 73
Amniocentesis, 7
Amputee, 11-12
Anderson, Ruth, 73
Apgar, Virginia, 6, 16, 181
Arthrogryposis, 12-13
Ataxia, 9
Athetosis, 9
Autonomy, in psychosexual development, 24, 211-212
(see also Effectance motivation, Separation from mother)
Awareness of other, 59, 66-67, 173-175, 179-180
Awkward gait, 4
Ayers, Jean, 137, 268

B

Barker, Roger, 6
Basic trust, sense of, 24, 29, 155
Beck, Joan, 6, 16, 181
Behavior modification, 217-219
Betthelheim, Bruno, 24, 155
Birth defects,
definition and etiology, 6-8
types, 8-14
Blindness, 5, 30
Bloom Benjamin S., 41, 44
Blount's Disease, 14
Body awareness, 59, 62, 159
techniques to enhance, 160
Bower, Eli, 219
Bowlby, John, 81
Bowleg, 14
Bracing, 11, 13, 14
Buhler, Charlotte, 24
Bzoch, Kenneth R., 71

Bzoch-League Receptive-Expressive Emergent Language Scale, 60, 71

C

Caplan, Gerald, 44
Casler, Lawrence, 30
Cattell Infant Scales, 36, 59-60, 72
Cattell, Psyche, 36, 72
Causality, concept of, 189-193
Cerebral palsy, 7, 8-9
characteristics, 8-9
etiology, 8
figure-ground disturbance in perception, 34
mental retardation in, 9, 31, 34, 261-269
motivation, 9
perceptual disorders in, 9, 181-182
speech disorders in, 9
types, 9, 31 (see also Spasticity, Ataxia, Athetosis)
Chromosomal disorders, 7-8
Circular reactions in sensorimotor period, 26-28
(see also Sensorimotor learning)
Classification, concepts of, 199-200
Cleveland Foundation, xiv
Clubfoot, 6, 11
Cognitive and affective interaction in development, 21, 33
Cognitive development, 21, 25-28
perennial issues in, 38
(see also Cognitive developmental curriculum, Concept learning)
Cognitive developmental curriculum, 188-209
Competence, sense of, 24, 186
(see also Effectance motivation)
Concept learning, 183-184, 208
conceptualization; role in development, 23, 25-28
(see also Cognitive development)

Congenital disorders, 12
  (*see also* Genetic factors)
Contractures, 9
Crabtree, Margaret, 71
Critical periods in development, 31, 38,
  41-42
Cruickshank, William M., 17, 34
Cystic fibrosis, 8

D

Deafness, 4, 5
Dennis, Wayne, 29
Deno, Evelyn S., 20
Diabetes, 7
Doll, Edgar A., 73
Dolphin, James E., 34
Down's Syndrome, 8

E

Eating Problems, 154-155
Education
  acceptance of handicapped children,
    19
  alternative approaches in program-
    ming, 19-20
  and social reform, 41
  architectural barriers, 18
  as prevention, 39, 43
  curriculum, 17, 188-209
  exclusion from school, 40
Effectance motivation, 24, 28-29, 150,
    162, 218-220
  (*see also* Competence, sense of)
Egocentrism in cognitive development,
    28, 185
Elkind, David, 25, 36
Emotional responses to handicapped
    persons, 4
Environmental factors in etiology, 11
Erikson, Erik H., 24, 38, 155, 211
Expressive language, 60, 71, 206-207

F

Fantz, Robert L., 22
Finnie, Nancie, 16, 135, 153
Fiorentino, Mary R., 133
Flavell, John, 188
Fraiberg, Selma, 30, 150
Freedheim, Donald K., 32

G

Genetic counseling, 7
Genetic disorders, 7
Genetic factors, 7, 11
  (*see also* Congenital disorders)
Gesell, Arnold L., 73
Gestalt School, 22
Gillette, Harriet E., 143
Ginsburg, Herbert, 35, 185
Gouin-Descaries, 30
Grouping of children, rationale for,
    167-168

H

Head Start, 18, 42
Hearing impairment, 4
Heart defect, 7
Hebb, Donald O., 41
Hemophilia, 7
Hospitalization, 150
  effects on psychological development,
    29-30
  (*see also* Maternal deprivation)
Houston Test for Language Development,
    60, 71
Hunt, J. McV., 35, 37, 41
Hydrocephalus, 7, 10-11
  (*see also* Shunting)

I

Ilg, Frances, 73
Illness
  encephalitis: 15
  high fever: 15
  meningitis: 15
  viral infection: 15
Imitation, role in cognitive develop-
    ment, 60, 67, 194-196, 206-207
Individuation, 81
  (*see also* Autonomy)
Inhelder, Barbel, 196, 200, 202
Intelligence of handicapped persons, 4,
    31, 34, 36-38
  effects of experience, 35, 41, 42
  measurement of, 31, 32, 34
Isaacs, Susan, 187

J

Johnson, G. Orville, 17
Juvenile rheumatoid arthritis, 13

K

Kamii, Constance, 203
Keats, Sidney, 9, 32
Kephart, Newell, 22
Kessen, William, 22
Kessler, Jane W., 33
Knobloch, Hilda, 73
Knock-knees, 14
    (*see also* Tibial torsion, Blount's Disease)

L

Language development, 23, 59-60, 194-199
    (*see also* Representation, Expressive language, Receptive language)
League, Richard, 71
Legg Calvé Perthes Disease, 14
Lehtinen, Laura E., 34
Lerrigo, Marion O., 16
Lewin, Kurt, 114
Limits, need for, 212-215
Logical thinking, development of, 185
    (*see also* Cognitive development)

M

Mahler, Margaret, 81, 151
Maternal deprivation, 30
    (*see also* Separation from mother)
Matheny, Patricia, 73
McGraw, Myrtle, 140, 143
McKay, R. James, 8, 9
Miles, Madeline, 73
Montessori, Maria, 182, 217
Motivation, 9, 217-221
    epistemic curiosity, 36
    function pleasure, 24
    intrinsic, 24
    (*see also* Effectance motivation)
Motor development, 23, 26, 30, 59, 72, 139-140
    (*see also* Physical therapy)
Myelodysplasia, 4, 7, 9-10
    characteristics, 10
    hydrocephalus in, 10
    incidence, 9
    myelomeningocele, 10
    (*see also* Spina bifida)

N

Najarian, P, 29
National Foundation/March of Dimes, 16
Negativism, 24, 217-221
Nelson, Waldo E., 8, 9
Nevis, Sonia, 22

O

Object concept, role in cognitive development, 25, 60, 69-70, 151, 157, 189-193
    in blind children, 30
    in thalidomide babies, 30
Occupational therapy, 59-60, 73, 143-145, 153-154
Ojemann, Ralph, 218
Opper, Sylvia, 35, 185
Orthopedic surgery, 11, 13
Osteogenesis imperfecta, 12

P

Page, Dorothy, 140
Parents of handicapped children, 80-113
    ambivalence and guilt, 50, 82-84, 86
    carry-over of habilitation program, 102-103, 104-113, 172, 223-225
    denial, 86-89
    family relations, 84, 89-95
    mothering experience, 81-84, 153
    need for feedback, 49
    need for support, 50, 84, 223-225
    overprotection, 86
    problems in separation, 85-86
    questions frequently asked, 95, 100-101, 103
    role of fathers, 90-94, 97
    role in rehabilitation, 58
    shock and grieving, 82, 100
    siblings, 81, 97-99
Passamanick, Benjamin, 73
Peer modeling, 176-177
Phelphs, William M., 31
Phocomelia, 12, 83
Physical therapy: 9, 13, 132-148, 152-153
    changing role: 132-134, 189-190
    gait training in: 11

integration with education: 134-139
sensory stimulation in: 158
Piaget, Jean, xii, 22, 25-28, 33, 35-38,
    114, 155, 185, 189, 194, 195, 196,
    200, 201, 202, 203, 218
    clinical method, 37
Pines, Maya, 43
Pinneau, Samuel R., 30
Plank, Emma, 150
Poison ingestion, 15
Powledge, Fred, 41
Preschool Attainment Record, 59-60, 72
Pressure sores, 9
Prosthesis with amputee, 11

R

Receptive language, stimulation of, 60,
    194-199
Reflex patterns in infant development,
    24, 25
    (*see also* Motor development)
Representation in cognitive develop-
    ment, 23, 149
    (*see also* Symbolic functioning, Cogni-
    tive development)
    Representation play
    (*see also* Sociodramatic play)
Rogers, Carl R., 29
Rohwer, William C., Jr., 38
Rubella, 7

S

Sattler, Jerome M., 32
Sawrey, James M., 9, 32
Self assertion, 156-157
Self-awareness, 59, 61-62, 149
Self-concept, 28-29, 44-45
Semans, Sarah, 133-134, 142
Sensory development in infancy, 22-23
    deprivation in infancy, 29-30
    in handicapped children, 29-31
    sensorimotor learning, 186-209
    sensorimotor schemata, 25-28, 37
    (*see also* Cognitive development)
Separation from mother, 169
Sherard, Earl, 73
Shunting, 10-11
Sickle cell anemia, 6
Sigel, Irving E., 26, 185

Silberman, Charles E., 39
Small, Gloria, 114
Smilansky, Sara, 161
Socialization as educational goal, 164-
    165
Society for Crippled Children, vii-ix,
    xiv, 16, 45, 96, 165
Sociodramatic play, 120, 161
    (*see also* Representation)
Spasticity, 9, 15, 132, 136
Special education, 17-20, 39-40
    inclusion of handicapped in regular
    education, 18-20
    (*see also* Education)
Spina bifida, 4, 9-10
    (*see also* Myelodysplasia)
Spitz, Rene A., 30, 81
Spock, Benjamin S., 16
State Bureau for the Handicapped, 15
Stockmeyer, Shirley A., 134, 139
Strauss, Alfred A., 34
Strauss Syndrome, 34
Sullivan, Harry S., 28, 151
Symbolic functioning, 23, 197-199
    (*see also* representation symbolic play)
Syphilis, 7

T

Tactile defensiveness, 137, 268
Tay-Sachs Disease, 6, 8
Teacher's Daily Record, 60, 74-77
Teacher's Periodic Checklist, 58-59, 60-71
Telford, Charles W., 9, 32
Textbook of Pediatrics, 8
Tibial torsion, 6, 14
    (*see also* Knock-knees)
Traditional beliefs concerning hand-
    icaps, 3
Tyler, Nancy S., 73

U

Uzgiris, Ina C., 37

V

Vaughan, Victor C., III, 8, 9
Verbalization in dealing with feelings,
    221-223
Vineland Social Maturity Scale, 59-60, 71,
    72

W

Wenar, Charles, 34
Weikart, David, 42

White, Robert W., 24, 218
Wolff, Peter H., 30
World Test, 34